# THE YOGA OF SELF-PERFECTION

## THE SYNTHESIS OF YOGA

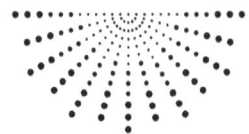

### SRI AUROBINDO

## CONTENTS

| | |
|---|---|
| The Principle of the Integral Yoga | 1 |
| The Integral Perfection | 7 |
| The Psychology of Self-Perfection | 14 |
| The Perfection of the Mental Being | 22 |
| The Instruments of the Spirit | 31 |
| Purification — The Lower Mentality | 41 |
| Purification — Intelligence and Will | 49 |
| The Liberation of the Spirit | 59 |
| The Liberation of the Nature | 67 |
| The Elements of Perfection | 75 |
| The Perfection of Equality | 81 |
| The Way of Equality | 90 |
| The Action of Equality | 101 |
| The Power of the Instruments | 108 |
| Soul-Force and the Fourfold Personality | 118 |
| The Divine Shakti | 129 |
| The Action of the Divine Shakti | 138 |
| Faith and Shakti | 146 |
| The Nature of the Supermind | 156 |
| The Intuitive Mind | 170 |
| The Gradations of the Supermind | 181 |
| The Supramental Thought and Knowledge | 194 |
| The Supramental Instruments — Thought-Process | 207 |
| The Supramental Sense | 226 |
| Towards the Supramental Time Vision | 246 |
| *Also by* SRI AUROBINDO | 263 |

# THE PRINCIPLE OF THE INTEGRAL YOGA

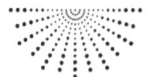

THE PRINCIPLE of Yoga is the turning of one or of all powers of our human existence into a means of reaching divine Being. In an ordinary Yoga one main power of being or one group of its powers is made the means, vehicle, path. In a synthetic Yoga all powers will be combined and included in the transmuting instrumentation.

In Hatha-yoga the instrument is the body and life. All the power of the body is stilled, collected, purified, heightened, concentrated to its utmost limits or beyond any limits by Asana and other physical processes; the power of the life too is similarly purified, heightened, concentrated by Asana and Pranayama. This concentration of powers is then directed towards that physical centre in which the divine consciousness sits concealed in the human body. The power of Life, Nature-power, coiled up with all its secret forces asleep in the lowest nervous plexus of the earth-being,—for only so much escapes into waking action in our normal operations as is sufficient for the limited uses of human life,— rises awakened through centre after centre and awakens, too, in its ascent and passage the forces of each successive nodus of our being, the nervous life, the heart of emotion and ordinary mentality, the speech, sight, will, the higher knowledge, till through and above the brain it meets with and it becomes one with the divine consciousness.

In Raja-yoga the chosen instrument is the mind. Our ordinary mentality is first disciplined, purified and directed towards the divine

Being, then by a summary process of Asana and Pranayama the physical force of our being is stilled and concentrated, the life-force released into a rhythmic movement capable of cessation and concentrated into a higher power of its upward action, the mind, supported and strengthened by this greater action and concentration of the body and life upon which it rests, is itself purified of all its unrest and emotion and its habitual thought-waves, liberated from distraction and dispersion, given its highest force of concentration, gathered up into a trance of absorption. Two objects, the one temporal, the other eternal, are gained by this discipline. Mind-power develops in another concentrated action abnormal capacities of knowledge, effective will, deep light of reception, powerful light of thought-radiation which are altogether beyond the narrow range of our normal mentality; it arrives at the Yogic or occult powers around which there has been woven so much quite dispensable and yet perhaps salutary mystery. But the one final end and the one all-important gain is that the mind, stilled and cast into a concentrated trance, can lose itself in the divine consciousness and the soul be made free to unite with the divine Being.

The triple way takes for its chosen instruments the three main powers of the mental soul-life of the human being. Knowledge selects the reason and the mental vision and it makes them by purification, concentration and a certain discipline of a God-directed seeking its means for the greatest knowledge and the greatest vision of all, God-knowledge and God-vision. Its aim is to see, know and be the Divine. Works, action selects for its instrument the will of the doer of works; it makes life an offering of sacrifice to the Godhead and by purification, concentration and a certain discipline of subjection to the divine Will a means for contact and increasing unity of the soul of man with the divine Master of the universe. Devotion selects the emotional and aesthetic powers of the soul and by turning them all Godward in a perfect purity, intensity, infinite passion of seeking makes them a means of God-possession in one or many relations of unity with the Divine Being. All aim in their own way at a union or unity of the human soul with the supreme Spirit.

Each Yoga in its process has the character of the instrument it uses; thus the Hatha-yogic process is psycho-physical, the Raja-yogic mental and psychic, the way of knowledge is spiritual and cognitive, the way of devotion spiritual, emotional and aesthetic, the way of works spiritual and dynamic by action. Each is guided in the ways of its own characteristic power. But all power is in the end one, all power is really soul-power. In the ordinary process of life, body and mind this truth is quite obscured by the dispersed, dividing and distributive action of Nature which is the normal condition of all our functionings, although even there it is in the end evident; for all material energy contains hidden the vital, mental, psychic, spiritual energy and in the end it must release these forms of the one Shakti, the vital energy conceals and liberates into action all the other forms, the mental supporting itself on the life and body and their powers and functionings contains undeveloped or only partially developed the psychic and the spiritual power of the being. But when by Yoga any of these powers is taken up from the dispersed and distributive action, raised to its highest degree, concentrated, it becomes manifest soul-power and reveals the essential unity. Therefore the Hatha-yogic process has too its pure psychic and spiritual result, the Raja-yogic arrives by psychic means at a spiritual consummation. The triple way may appear to be altogether mental and spiritual in its way of seeking and its objectives, but it can be attended by results more characteristic of the other paths, which offer themselves in a spontaneous and involuntary flowering, and for the same reason, because soul-power is all-power and where it reaches its height in one direction its other possibilities also begin to show themselves in fact or in incipient potentiality. This unity at once suggests the possibility of a synthetic Yoga.

Tantric discipline is in its nature a synthesis. It has seized on the large universal truth that there are two poles of being whose essential unity is the secret of existence, Brahman and Shakti, Spirit and Nature, and that Nature is power of the spirit or rather is spirit as power. To raise nature in man into manifest power of spirit is its method and it is the whole nature that it gathers up for the spiritual conversion. It includes in its system of instrumentation the forceful Hatha-yogic process and especially the opening up of the nervous centres and the passage through them of the awakened Shakti on her way to her union with the Brahman, the subtler stress of the Raja-yogic purification, meditation and concentration, the leverage of will-force, the motive power of devotion, the key of knowledge. But it does not stop short with an effective assembling of the different powers of these specific Yogas. In two directions it enlarges by its synthetic turn the province of the Yogic method. First, it lays its hand firmly on many of the main springs of human quality, desire, action and it subjects them to an intensive discipline with the soul's mastery of its motives as a first aim and their elevation to a diviner spiritual level as its final utility. Again, it includes in its objects of Yoga not only liberation,[1] which is the one all-mastering preoccupation of the specific systems, but a cosmic enjoyment[2] of the power of the Spirit, which the others may take incidentally on the way, in part, casually, but avoid making a motive or object. It is a bolder and larger system.

In the method of synthesis which we have been following, another clue of principle has been pursued which is derived from another view of the possibilities of Yoga. This starts from the method of Vedanta to arrive at the aim of the Tantra. In the Tantric method Shakti is all-important, becomes the key to the finding of spirit; in this synthesis spirit, soul is all-important, becomes the secret of the taking up of Shakti. The Tantric method starts from the bottom and grades the ladder of ascent upwards to the summit; therefore its initial stress is upon the action of the awakened Shakti in the nervous system of the body and its centres; the opening of the six lotuses is the opening up of the ranges of the power of Spirit. Our synthesis takes man as a spirit in mind much more than a spirit in body and assumes in him the capacity to begin on that level, to spiritualise his being by the power of the soul in mind opening itself directly to a higher spiritual force and being and to perfect by that higher force so possessed and brought into action the whole of his nature. For that reason our initial stress has fallen upon the utilisation of the powers of soul in mind and the turning of the triple key of knowledge, works and love in the locks of the spirit; the Hatha-yogic methods can be dispensed with,—though there is no objection to their partial use, —the Raja-yogic will only enter in as an informal element. To arrive by the shortest way at the largest development of spiritual power and being and divinise by it a liberated nature in the whole range of human living is our inspiring motive.

The principle in view is a self-surrender, a giving up of the human being into the being, consciousness, power, delight of the Divine, a union or communion at all the points of meeting in the soul of man, the mental being, by which the Divine himself, directly and without veil master and possessor of the instrument, shall by the light of his presence and guidance perfect the human being in all the forces of the Nature for a divine living. Here we arrive at a farther enlargement of the objects of the Yoga. The common initial purpose of all Yoga is the liberation of the soul of man from its present natural ignorance and limitation, its release into spiritual being, its union with the highest self and Divinity. But ordinarily this is made not only the initial but the whole and final object: enjoyment of spiritual being there is, but either in a dissolution of the human and individual into the silence of self-being or on a higher plane in another existence. The Tantric system makes liberation the final, but not the only aim; it takes on its way a full perfection and enjoyment of the spiritual power, light and joy in the human existence, and even it has a glimpse of a supreme experience in which liberation and cosmic action and enjoyment are unified in a final overcoming of all oppositions and dissonances. It is this wider view of our spiritual potentialities from which we begin, but we add another stress which brings in a completer significance. We regard the spirit in man not as solely an individual being travelling to a transcendent unity with the Divine, but as a universal being capable of oneness with the Divine in all souls and all Nature and we give this extended view its entire practical consequence. The human soul's individual liberation and enjoyment of union with the Divine in spiritual being, consciousness and delight must always be the first object of the Yoga; its free enjoyment of the cosmic unity of the Divine becomes a second object; but out of that a third appears, the effectuation of the meaning of the divine unity with all beings by a sympathy and participation in the spiritual purpose of the Divine in humanity. The individual Yoga then turns from its separateness and becomes a part of the collective Yoga of the divine Nature in the human race. The liberated individual being, united with the Divine in self and spirit, becomes in his natural being a self-perfecting instrument for the perfect out-flowering of the Divine in humanity.

This out-flowering has its two terms; first, comes the growth out of the separative human ego into the unity of the spirit, then the possession of the divine nature in its proper and its higher forms and no longer in the inferior forms of the mental being which are a mutilated translation and not the authentic text of the original script of divine Nature in the cosmic individual. In other words, a perfection has to be aimed at which amounts to the elevation of the mental into the full spiritual and supramental nature. Therefore this integral Yoga of knowledge, love and works has to be extended into a Yoga of spiritual and gnostic self-perfection. As gnostic knowledge, will and ananda are a direct instrumentation of spirit and can only be won by growing into the spirit, into divine being, this growth has to be the first aim of our Yoga. The mental being has to enlarge itself into the oneness of the Divine before the Divine will perfect in the soul of the individual its gnostic out-flowering. That is the reason why the triple way of knowledge, works and love becomes the key-note of the whole Yoga, for that is the direct means for the soul in mind to rise to its highest intensities where it passes upward into the divine oneness. That too is the reason why the Yoga must be integral. For if immergence in the Infinite or some close union with the Divine were all our aim, an integral Yoga would be superfluous, except for such greater satisfaction of the being of man as we may get by a self-lifting of the whole of it towards its Source. But it would not be needed for the essential aim, since by any single power of the soul-nature we can meet with the Divine; each at its height rises up into the infinite and absolute, each therefore offers a sufficient way of arrival, for all the hundred separate paths meet in the Eternal. But the gnostic being is a complete enjoyment and possession of the whole divine and spiritual nature; and it is a complete lifting of the whole nature of man into its power of a divine and spiritual existence. Integrality becomes then an essential condition of this Yoga.

At the same time we have seen that each of the three ways at its height, if it is pursued with a certain largeness, can take into itself the powers of the others and lead to their fulfillment. It is therefore sufficient to start by one of them and find the point at which it meets the other at first parallel lines of advance and melts into them by its own widenings. At the same time a more difficult, complex, wholly powerful process would be to start, as it were, on three lines together, on a triple wheel of soul-power. But the consideration of this possibility must be postponed till we have seen what are the conditions and means of the Yoga of self-perfection. For we shall see that this also need not be postponed entirely, but a certain preparation of it is part of and a certain initiation into it proceeds by the growth of the divine works, love and knowledge.

---

1. Mukti.
2. Bhukti.

# THE INTEGRAL PERFECTION

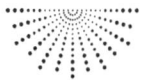

A DIVINE perfection of the human being is our aim. We must know then first what are the essential elements that constitute man's total perfection; secondly, what we mean by a divine as distinguished from a human perfection of our being. That man as a being is capable of self-development and of some approach at least to an ideal standard of perfection which his mind is able to conceive, fix before it and pursue, is common ground to all thinking humanity, though it may be only the minority who concern themselves with this possibility as providing the one most important aim of life. But by some the ideal is conceived as a mundane change, by others as a religious conversion.

The mundane perfection is sometimes conceived of as something outward, social, a thing of action, a more rational dealing with our fellow-men and our environment, a better and more efficient citizenship and discharge of duties, a better, richer, kindlier and happier way of living, with a more just and more harmonious associated enjoyment of the opportunities of existence. By others again a more inner and subjective ideal is cherished, a clarifying and raising of the intelligence, will and reason, a heightening and ordering of power and capacity in the nature, a nobler ethical, a richer aesthetic, a finer emotional, a much healthier and better-governed vital and physical being. Sometimes one element is stressed, almost to the exclusion of the rest; sometimes, in wider and more well-balanced minds, the whole harmony is envisaged as a total perfection. A change of education and social institutions is the outward means adopted or an inner self-training and development is preferred as the true instrumentation. Or the two aims may be clearly united, the perfection of the inner individual, the perfection of the outer living.

But the mundane aim takes for its field the present life and its opportunities; the religious aim on the contrary fixes before it the self-preparation for another existence after death, its commonest ideal is some kind of pure sainthood, its means a conversion of the imperfect or sinful human being by divine grace or through obedience to a law laid down by a scripture or else given by a religious founder. The aim of religion may include a social change, but it is then a change brought about by the acceptance of a common religious ideal and way of consecrated living, a brotherhood of the saints, a theocracy or kingdom of God reflecting on earth the kingdom of heaven.

The object of our synthetic Yoga must, in this respect too as in its other parts, be more integral and comprehensive, embrace all these elements or these tendencies of a larger impulse of self-perfection and harmonise them or rather unify, and in order to do that successfully it must seize on a truth which is wider than the ordinary religious and higher than the mundane principle. All life is a secret Yoga, an obscure growth of Nature towards the discovery and fulfilment of the divine principle hidden in her which becomes progressively less obscure, more self-conscient and luminous, more self-possessed in the human being by the opening of all his instruments of knowledge, will, action, life to the Spirit within him and in the world. Mind, life, body, all the forms of our nature are the means of this growth, but they find their last perfection only by opening out to something beyond them, first, because they are not the whole of what man is, secondly, because that other something which he is, is the key of his completeness and brings a light which discovers to him the whole high and large reality of his being.

Mind is fulfilled by a greater knowledge of which it is only a half-light, life discovers its meaning in a greater power and will of which it is the outward and as yet obscure functioning, body finds its last use as an instrument of a power of being of which it is a physical support and material starting-point. They have all themselves first to be developed and find out their ordinary possibilities; all our normal life is a trying of these possibilities and an opportunity for this preparatory and tentative self-training. But life cannot find its perfect self-fulfilment till it opens to that greater reality of being of which by this development of a richer power and a more sensitive use and capacity it becomes a well-prepared field of working.

Intellectual, volitional, ethical, emotional, aesthetic and physical training and improvement are all so much to the good, but they are only in the end a constant movement in a circle without any last delivering and illumining aim, unless they arrive at a point when they can open themselves to the power and presence of the Spirit and admit its direct workings. This direct working effects a conversion of the whole being which is the indispensable condition of our real perfection. To grow into the truth and power of the Spirit and by the direct action of that power to be made a fit channel of its self-expression,—a living of man in the Divine and a divine living of the Spirit in humanity,—will therefore be the principle and the whole object of an integral Yoga of self-perfection.

In the process of this change there must be by the very necessity of the effort two stages of its working. First, there will be the personal endeavour of the human being, as soon as he becomes aware by his soul, mind, heart of this divine possibility and turns towards it as the true object of life, to prepare himself for it and to get rid of all in him that belongs to a lower working, of all that stands in the way of his opening to the spiritual truth and its power, so as to possess by this liberation his spiritual being and turn all his natural movements into free means of its self-expression. It is by this turn that the self-conscious Yoga aware of its aim begins: there is a new awakening and an upward change of the life motive. So long as there is only an intellectual, ethical and other self-training for the now normal purposes of life which does not travel beyond the ordinary circle of working of mind, life and body, we are still only in the obscure and yet unillumined preparatory Yoga of Nature; we are still in pursuit of only an ordinary human perfection. A spiritual desire of the Divine and of the divine perfection, of a unity with him in all our being and a spiritual perfection in all our nature, is the effective sign of this change, the precursory power of a great integral conversion of our being and living.

By personal effort a precursory change, a preliminary conversion can be effected; it amounts to a greater or less spiritualising of our mental motives, our character and temperament, and a mastery, stilling or changed action of the vital and physical life. This converted subjectivity can be made the base of some communion or unity of the soul in mind with the Divine and some partial reflection of the divine nature in the mentality of the human being. That is as far as man can go by his unaided or indirectly aided effort, because that is an effort of mind and mind cannot climb beyond itself permanently: at most it arises to a spiritualised and idealised mentality. If it shoots up beyond that border, it loses hold of itself, loses hold of life, and arrives either at a trance of absorption or a passivity. A greater perfection can only be arrived at by a higher power entering in and taking up the whole action of the being. The second stage of this Yoga will therefore be a persistent giving up of all the action of the nature into the hands of this greater Power, a substitution of its influence, possession and working for the personal effort, until the Divine to whom we aspire becomes the direct master of the Yoga and effects the entire spiritual and ideal conversion of the being.

This double character of our Yoga raises it beyond the mundane ideal of perfection, while at the same time it goes too beyond the loftier, intenser, but much narrower religious formula. The mundane ideal regards man always as a mental, vital and physical being and it aims at a human perfection well within these limits, a perfection of mind, life and body, an expansion and refinement of the intellect and knowledge, of the will and power, of ethical character, aim and conduct, of aesthetic sensibility and creativeness, of emotional balanced poise and enjoyment, of vital and physical soundness, regulated action and just efficiency. It is a wide and full aim, but yet not sufficiently full and wide, because it ignores that other greater element of our being which the mind vaguely conceives as the spiritual element and leaves it either undeveloped or insufficiently satisfied as merely some high occasional or added derivatory experience, the result of the action of mind in its exceptional aspects or dependent upon mind for its presence and persistence. It can become a high aim when it seeks to develop the loftier and the larger reaches of our mentality, but yet not sufficiently high, because it does not aspire beyond mind to that of which our purest reason, our brightest mental intuition, our deepest mental sense and feeling, strongest mental will and power or ideal aim and purpose are only pale radiations. Its aim besides is limited to a terrestrial perfection of the normal human life.

A Yoga of integral perfection regards man as a divine spiritual being involved in mind, life and body; it aims therefore at a liberation and a perfection of his divine nature. It seeks to make an inner living in the perfectly developed spiritual being his constant intrinsic living and the spiritualised action of mind, life and body only its outward human expression. In order that this spiritual being may not be something vague and indefinable or else but imperfectly realised and dependent on the mental support and the mental limitations, it seeks to go beyond mind to the supramental knowledge, will, sense, feeling, intuition, dynamic initiation of vital and physical action, all that makes the native working of the spiritual being. It accepts human life, but takes account of the large supraterrestrial action behind the earthly material living, and it joins itself to the divine Being from whom the supreme origination of all these partial and lower states proceeds so that the whole of life may become aware of its divine source and feel in each action of knowledge, of will, of feeling, sense and body the divine originating impulse. It rejects nothing that is essential in the mundane aim, but enlarges it, finds and lives in its greater and its truer meaning now hidden from it, transfigures it from a limited, earthly and mortal thing to a figure of infinite, divine and immortal values.

The integral Yoga meets the religious ideal at several points, but goes beyond it in the sense of a greater wideness. The religious ideal looks, not only beyond this earth, but away from it to a heaven or even beyond all heavens to some kind of Nirvana. Its ideal of perfection is limited to whatever kind of inner or outer mutation will eventually serve the turning away of the soul from the human life to the beyond. Its ordinary idea of perfection is a religio-ethical change, a drastic purification of the active and the emotional being, often with an ascetic abrogation and rejection of the vital impulses as its completest reaching of excellence, and in any case a supraterrestrial motive and reward or result of a life of piety and right conduct. In so far as it admits a change of knowledge, will, aesthesis, it is in the sense of the turning of them to another object than the aims of human life and eventually brings a rejection of all earthly objects of aesthesis, will and knowledge. The method, whether it lays stress on personal effort or upon divine influence, on works and knowledge or upon grace, is not like the mundane a development, but rather a conversion; but in the end the aim is not a conversion of our mental and physical nature, but the putting on of a pure spiritual nature and being, and since that is not possible here on earth, it looks for its consummation by a transference to another world or a shuffling off of all cosmic existence.

But the integral Yoga founds itself on a conception of the spiritual being as an omnipresent existence, the fullness of which comes not essentially by a transference to other worlds or a cosmic self-extinction, but by a growth out of what we now are phenomenally into the consciousness of the omnipresent reality which we always are in the essence of our being. It substitutes for the form of religious piety its completer spiritual seeking of a divine union. It proceeds by a personal effort to a conversion through a divine influence and possession; but this divine grace, if we may so call it, is not simply a mysterious flow or touch coming from above, but the all-pervading act of a divine presence which we come to know within as the power of the highest Self and Master of our being entering into the soul and so possessing it that we not only feel it close to us and pressing upon our mortal nature, but live in its law, know that law, possess it as the whole power of our spiritualised nature. The conversion its action will effect is an integral conversion of our ethical being into the Truth and Right of the divine nature, of our intellectual into the illumination of divine knowledge, our emotional into the divine love and unity, our dynamic and volitional into a working of the divine power, our aesthetic into a plenary reception and a creative enjoyment of divine beauty, not excluding even in the end a divine conversion of the vital and physical being. It regards all the previous life as an involuntary and unconscious or half-conscious preparatory growing towards this change and Yoga as the voluntary and conscious effort and realisation of the change, by which all the aim of human existence in all its parts is fulfilled, even while it is transfigured. Admitting the supracosmic truth and life in worlds beyond, it admits to the terrestrial as a continued term of the one existence and a change of individual and communal life on earth as a strain of its divine meaning.

To open oneself to the supracosmic Divine is an essential condition of this integral perfection; to unite oneself with the universal Divine is another essential condition. Here the Yoga of self-perfection coincides with the Yogas of knowledge, works and devotion; for it is impossible to change the human nature into the divine or to make it an instrument of the divine knowledge, will and joy of existence, unless there is a union with the supreme Being, Consciousness and Bliss and a unity with its universal Self in all things and beings. A wholly separative possession of the divine nature by the human individual, as distinct from a self-withdrawn absorption in it, is not possible. But this unity will not be an inmost spiritual oneness qualified, so long as the human life lasts, by a separative existence in mind, life and body; the full perfection is a possession, through this spiritual unity, of unity too with the universal Mind, the universal Life, the universal Form which are the other constant terms of cosmic being. Moreover, since human life is still accepted as a self-expression of the realised Divine in man, there must be an action of the entire divine nature in our life; and this brings in the need of the supramental conversion which substitutes the native action of spiritual being for the imperfect action of the superficial nature and spiritualises and transfigures its mental, vital and physical parts by the spiritual ideality. These three elements, a union with the supreme Divine, unity with the universal Self, and a supramental life action from this transcendent origin and through this universality, but still with the individual as the soul-channel and natural instrument, constitute the essence of the integral divine perfection of the human being.

# THE PSYCHOLOGY OF SELF-PERFECTION

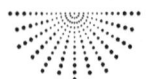

ESSENTIALLY, then, this divine self-perfection is a conversion of the human into a likeness of and a fundamental oneness with the divine nature, a rapid shaping of the image of God in man and filling in of its ideal outlines. It is what is ordinarily termed *sādṛśya-mukti*, a liberation into the divine resemblance out of the bondage of the human seeming, or, to use the expression of the Gita, *sādharmya-gati*, a coming to be one in law of being with the supreme, universal and indwelling Divine. To perceive and have a right view of our way to such a transformation we must form some sufficient working idea of the complex thing that this human nature at present is in the confused interminglings of its various principles, so that we may see the precise nature of the conversion each part of it must undergo and the most effective means for the conversion. How to disengage from this knot of thinking mortal matter the Immortal it contains, from this mentalised vital animal man the happy fullness of his submerged hints of Godhead, is the real problem of a human being and living. Life develops many first hints of the divinity without completely disengaging them; Yoga is the unravelling of the knot of Life's difficulty.

First of all we have to know the central secret of the psychological complexity which creates the problem and all its difficulties. But an ordinary psychology which only takes mind and its phenomena at their surface values, will be of no help to us; it will not give us the least guidance in this line of self-exploration and self-conversion. Still less can we find the clue in a scientific psychology with a materialistic basis which assumes that the body and the biological and physiological factors of our nature are not only the starting-point but the whole real foundation and regards human mind as only a subtle development from the life and the body. That may be the actual truth of the animal side of human nature and of the human mind in so far as it is limited and conditioned by the physical part of our being. But the whole difference between man and the animal is that the animal mind, as we know it, cannot get for one moment away from its origins, cannot break out from the covering, the close chrysalis which the bodily life has spun round the soul, and become something greater than its present self, a more free, magnificent and noble being; but in man mind reveals itself as a greater energy escaping from the restrictions of the vital and physical formula of being. But even this is not all that man is or can be: he has in him the power to evolve and release a still greater ideal energy which in its turn escapes out of the restrictions of the mental formula of his nature and discloses the supramental form, the ideal power of a spiritual being. In Yoga we have to travel beyond the physical nature and the superficial man and to discover the workings of the whole nature of the real man. In other words we must arrive at and use a psycho-physical knowledge with a spiritual foundation.

Man is in his real nature,—however obscure now this truth may be to our present understanding and self-consciousness, we must for the purposes of Yoga have faith in it, and we shall then find that our faith is justified by an increasing experience and a greater self-knowledge,—a spirit using the mind, life and body for an individual and a communal experience and self-manifestation in the universe. This spirit is an infinite existence limiting itself in apparent being for individual experience. It is an infinite consciousness which defines itself in finite forms of consciousness for joy of various knowledge and various power of being. It is an infinite delight of being expanding and contracting itself and its powers, concealing and discovering, formulating many terms of its joy of existence, even to an apparent obscuration and denial of its own nature. In itself it is eternal Sachchidananda, but this complexity, this knotting up and unravelling of the infinite in the finite is the aspect we see it assume in universal and in individual nature. To discover the eternal Sachchidananda, this essential self of our being within us, and live in it is the stable basis, to make its true nature evident and creative of a divine way of living in our instruments, supermind, mind, life and body, the active principle of a spiritual perfection.

Supermind, mind, life and body are the four instruments which the spirit uses for its manifestation in the workings of Nature. Supermind is spiritual consciousness acting as a self-luminous knowledge, will, sense, aesthesis, energy, self-creative and unveiling power of its own delight and being. Mind is the action of the same powers, but limited and only very indirectly and partially illumined. Supermind lives in unity though it plays with diversity; mind lives in a separative action of diversity, though it may open to unity. Mind is not only capable of ignorance, but, because it acts always partially and by limitation, it works characteristically as a power of ignorance: it may even and it does forget itself in a complete inconscience, or nescience, awaken from it to the ignorance of a partial knowledge and move from the ignorance towards a complete knowledge,—that is its natural action in the human being,—but it can never have by itself a complete knowledge. Supermind is incapable of real ignorance; even if it puts full knowledge behind it in the limitation of a particular working, yet all its working refers back to what it has put behind it and all is instinct with self-illumination; even if it involves itself in material nescience, it yet does there accurately the works of a perfect will and knowledge. Supermind lends itself to the action of the inferior instruments; it is always there indeed at the core as a secret support of their operations. In matter it is an automatic action and effectuation of the hidden idea in things; in life its most seizable form is instinct, an instinctive, subconscious or partly subconscious knowledge and operation; in mind it reveals itself as intuition, a swift, direct and self-effective illumination of intelligence, will, sense and aesthesis. But these are merely irradiations of the supermind which accommodate themselves to the limited functioning of the obscurer instruments: its own characteristic nature is a gnosis superconscient to mind, life and body. Supermind or gnosis is the characteristic, illumined, significant action of spirit in its own native reality.

Life is an energy of spirit subordinated to action of mind and body, which fulfils itself through mentality and physicality and acts as a link between them. It has its own characteristic operation but nowhere works independently of mind and body. All energy of the spirit in action works in the two terms of existence and consciousness, for the self-formation of existence and the play and self-realisation of consciousness, for the delight of existence and the delight of consciousness. In this inferior formulation of being in which we at present live, the spirit's energy of life works between the two terms of mind and matter, supporting and effecting the formulations of substance of matter and working as a material energy, supporting the formulations of consciousness of mind and the workings of mental energy, supporting the interaction of mind and body and working as a sensory and nervous energy. What we call vitality is for the purposes of our normal human existence power of conscious being emerging in matter, liberating from it and in it mind and the higher powers and supporting their limited action in the physical life,—just as what we call mentality is power of conscious being awaking in body to light of its own consciousness and to consciousness of all the rest of being immediately around it and working at first in the limited action set for it by life and body, but at certain points and at a certain height escaping from it to a partial action beyond this circle. But this is not the whole power whether of life or mentality; they have planes of conscious existence of their own kind, other than this material level, where they are freer in their characteristic action. Matter or body itself is a limiting form of substance of spirit in which life and mind and spirit are involved, self-hidden, self-forgetful by absorption in their own externalising action, but bound to emerge from it by a self-compelling evolution. But matter too is capable of refining to subtler forms of substance in which it becomes more apparently a formal density of life, of mind, of spirit. Man himself has, besides this gross material body, an encasing vital sheath, a mental body, a body of bliss and gnosis. But all matter, all body contains within it the secret powers of these higher principles; matter is a formation of life that has no real existence apart from the informing universal spirit which gives it its energy and substance.

This is the nature of spirit and its instruments. But to understand its operations and to get at a knowledge which will give to us a power of leverage in uplifting them out of the established groove in which our life goes spinning, we have to perceive that the Spirit has based all its workings upon two twin aspects of its being, Soul and Nature, Purusha and Prakriti. We have to treat them as different and diverse in power,—for in practice of consciousness this difference is valid,—although they are only two sides of the same reality, pole and pole of the one conscious being. Purusha or soul is spirit cognizant of the workings of its nature, supporting them by its being, enjoying or rejecting enjoyment of them in its delight of being. Nature is power of the spirit, and she is too working and process of its power formulating name and form of being, developing action of consciousness and knowledge, throwing itself up in will and impulsion, force and energy, fulfilling itself in enjoyment. Nature is Prakriti, Maya, Shakti. If we look at her on her most external side where she seems the opposite of Purusha, she is Prakriti, an inert and mechanical self-driven operation, inconscient or conscient only by the light of Purusha, elevated by various degrees, vital, mental, supramental, of his soul-illumination of her workings. If we look at her on her other internal side where she moves nearer to unity with Purusha, she is Maya, will of being and becoming or of cessation from being and becoming with all their results, apparent to the consciousness, of involution and evolution, existing and non-existing, self-concealment of spirit and self-discovery of spirit. Both are sides of one and the same thing, Shakti, power of being of the spirit which operates, whether superconsciously or consciously or subconsciously in a seeming inconscience,—in fact all these motions coexist at the same time and in the same soul,—as the spirit's power of knowledge, power of will, power of process and action, *jñāna- śakti, icchā-śakti, kriyā-śakti*. By this power the spirit creates all things in itself, hides and discovers all itself in the form and behind the veil of its manifestation.

Purusha is able by this power of its nature to take whatever poise it may will and to follow the law and form of being proper to any self-formulation. It is eternal soul and spirit in its own power of self-existence superior to and governing its manifestations; it is universal soul and spirit developed in power of becoming of its existence, infinite in the finite; it is individual soul and spirit absorbed in development of some particular course of its becoming, in appearance mutably finite in the infinite. All these things it can be at once, eternal spirit universalised in cosmos, individualised in its beings; it can too found the consciousness rejecting, governing or responding to the action of Nature in any one of them, put the others behind it or away from it, know itself as pure eternity, self-supporting universality or exclusive individuality. Whatever the formulation of its nature, soul can seem to become that and view itself as that only in the frontal active part of its consciousness; but it is never only what it seems to be; it is too the so much else that it can be; secretly, it is the all of itself that is yet hidden. It is not irrevocably limited by any particular self-formulation in Time, but can break through and beyond it, break it up or develop it, select, reject, new-create, reveal out of itself a greater self-formulation. What it believes itself to be by the whole active will of its consciousness in its instruments, that it is or tends to become, *yo yacchraddhaḥ sa eva saḥ* : what it believes it can be and has full faith in becoming, that it changes to in nature, evolves or discovers.

This power of the soul over its nature is of the utmost importance in the Yoga of self-perfection; if it did not exist, we could never get by conscious endeavour and aspiration out of the fixed groove of our present imperfect human being; if any greater perfection were intended, we should have to wait for Nature to effect it in her own slow or swift process of evolution. In the lower forms of being the soul accepts this complete subjection to Nature, but as it rises higher in the scale, it awakes to a sense of something in itself which can command Nature; but it is only when it arrives at self-knowledge that this free will and control becomes a complete reality. The change effects itself through process of nature, not therefore by any capricious magic, but an ordered development and intelligible process. When complete mastery is gained, then the process by its self-effective rapidity may seem a miracle to the intelligence, but it still proceeds by law of the truth of Spirit,—when the Divine within us by close union of our will and being with him takes up the Yoga and acts as the omnipotent master of the nature. For the Divine is our highest Self and the self of all Nature, the eternal and universal Purusha.

Purusha may establish himself in any plane of being, take any principle of being as the immediate head of his power and live in the working of its proper mode of conscious action. The soul may dwell in the principle of infinite unity of self-existence and be aware of all consciousness, energy, delight, knowledge, will, activity as conscious form of this essential truth, Sat or Satya. It may dwell in the principle of infinite conscious energy, Tapas, and be aware of it unrolling out of self-existence the works of knowledge, will and dynamic soul-action for the enjoyment of an infinite delight of the being. It may dwell in the principle of infinite self-existent delight and be aware of the divine Ananda creating out of its self-existence by its energy whatever harmony of being. In these three poises the consciousness of unity dominates; the soul lives in its awareness of eternity, universality, unity, and whatever diversity there is, is not separative, but only a multitudinous aspect of oneness. It may dwell too in the principle of supermind, in a luminous self-determining knowledge, will and action which develops some coordination of perfect delight of conscious being. In the higher gnosis unity is the basis, but it takes its joy in diversity; in lower fact of supermind diversity is the basis, but it refers back always to a conscious unity and it takes joy in unity. These ranges of consciousness are beyond our present level; they are superconscious to our normal mentality. That belongs to a lower hemisphere of being.

This lower being begins where a veil falls between soul and nature, between spirit in supermind and spirit in mind, life and body. Where this veil has not fallen, these instrumental powers are not what they are in us, but an enlightened part of the unified action of supermind and spirit. Mind gets to an independent idea of its own action when it forgets to refer back to the light from which it derives and becomes absorbed in the possibilities of its own separative process and enjoyment. The soul when it dwells in the principle of mind, not yet subject to but user of life and body, knows itself as a mental being working out its mental life and forces and images, bodies of the subtle mental substance, according to its individual knowledge, will and dynamis modified by its relation to other similar beings and powers in the universal mind. When it dwells in the principle of life, it knows itself as a being of the universal life working out action and consciousness by its desires under similar modifying conditions proper to a universal life-soul whose action is through many individual life-beings. When it dwells in the principle of matter, it knows itself as a consciousness of matter acting under a similar law of the energy of material being. In proportion as it leans towards the side of knowledge, it is aware of itself more or less clearly as a soul of mind, a soul of life, a soul of body viewing and acting in or acted upon by its nature; but where it leans towards the side of ignorance, it knows itself as an ego identified with nature of mind, of life or of body, a creation of Nature. But the native tendency of material being leads towards an absorption of the soul's energy in the act of formation and material movement and a consequent self-oblivion of the conscious being. The material universe begins from an apparent inconscience.

The universal Purusha dwells in all these planes in a certain simultaneity and builds upon each of these principles a world or series of worlds with its beings who live in the nature of that principle. Man, the microcosm, has all these planes in his own being, ranged from his subconscient to his superconscient existence. By a developing power of Yoga he can become aware of these concealed worlds hidden from his physical, materialised mind and senses which know only the material world, and then he becomes aware that his material existence is not a thing apart and self-existent, as the material universe in which he lives is also not a thing apart and self-existent, but is in constant relation to the higher planes and acted on by their powers and beings. He can open up and increase the action of these higher planes in himself and enjoy some sort of participation in the life of the other worlds,—which, for the rest, are or can be his dwelling-place, that is to say, the station of his awareness, *dhāma*, after death or between death and rebirth in a material body. But his most important capacity is that of developing the powers of the higher principles in himself, a greater power of life, a purer light of mind, the illumination of supermind, the infinite being, consciousness and delight of spirit. By an ascending movement he can develop his human imperfection towards that greater perfection.

But whatever his aim, however exalted his aspiration, he has to begin from the law of his present imperfection, to take full account of it and see how it can be converted to the law of a possible perfection. This present law of his being starts from the inconscience of the material universe, an involution of the soul in form and subjection to material nature; and, though in this matter life and mind have developed their own energies, yet they are limited and bound up in the action of the lower material, which is to the ignorance of his practical surface consciousness his original principle. Mind in him, though he is an embodied mental being, has to bear the control of the body and the physical life and can only by some more or less considerable effort of energy and concentration consciously control life and body. It is only by increasing that control that he can move towards perfection,—and it is only by developing soul-power that he can reach it. Nature-power in him has to become more and more completely a conscious act of soul, a conscious expression of all the will and knowledge of spirit. Prakriti has to reveal itself as shakti of the Purusha.

# THE PERFECTION OF THE MENTAL BEING

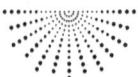

THE FUNDAMENTAL idea of a Yoga of self-perfection must be, under these conditions, a reversal of the present relations of the soul of man to his mental, vital and physical nature. Man is at present a partly self-conscious soul subject to and limited by mind, life and body, who has to become an entirely self-conscious soul master of his mind, life and body. Not limited by their claims and demands, a perfect self-conscious soul would be superior to and a free possessor of its instruments. This effort of man to be master of his own being has been the sense of a large part of his past spiritual, intellectual and moral strivings.

In order to be possessor of his being with any complete reality of freedom and mastery, man must find out his highest self, the real man or highest Purusha in him, which is free and master in its own inalienable power. He must cease to be the mental, vital, physical ego; for that is always the creation, instrument and subject of mental, vital, physical Nature. This ego is not his real self, but an instrumentation of Nature by which it has developed a sense of limited and separate individual being in mind, life and body. By this instrumentation he acts as if he were a separate existence in the material universe. Nature has evolved certain habitual limiting conditions under which that action takes place; self-identification of the soul with the ego is the means by which she induces the soul to consent to this action and accept these habitual limiting conditions. While the identification lasts, there is a self-imprisonment in this habitual round and narrow action, and, until it is transcended, there can be no free use by the soul of its individual living, much less a real self-exceeding. For this reason an essential movement of the Yoga is to draw back from the outward ego sense by which we are identified with the action of mind, life and body and live inwardly in the soul. The liberation from an externalised ego sense is the first step towards the soul's freedom and mastery.

When we thus draw back into the soul, we find ourselves to be not the mind, but a mental being who stands behind the action of the embodied mind, not a mental and vital personality,—personality is a composition of Nature,—but a mental Person, *manomaya puruṣa*. We become aware of a being within who takes his stand upon mind for self-knowledge and world-knowledge and thinks of himself as an individual for self-experience and world-experience, for an inward action and an outward-going action, but is yet different from mind, life and body. This sense of difference from the vital actions and the physical being is very marked; for although the Purusha feels his mind to be involved in life and body, yet he is aware that even if the physical life and body were to cease or be dissolved, he would still go on existing in his mental being. But the sense of difference from the mind is more difficult and less firmly distinct. But still it is there; it is characterised by any or all of three intuitions in which this mental Purusha lives and becomes by them aware of his own greater existence.

First, he has the intuition of himself as someone observing the action of the mind; it is something which is going on in him and yet before him as an object of his regarding knowledge. This self-awareness is the intuitive sense of the witness Purusha, *sākṣī*. Witness Purusha is a pure consciousness who watches Nature and sees it as an action reflected upon the consciousness and enlightened by that consciousness, but in itself other than it. To mental Purusha Nature is only an action, a complex action of discriminating and combining thought, of will, of sense, of emotion, of temperament and character, of ego feeling, which works upon a foundation of vital impulses, needs and cravings in the conditions imposed by the physical body. But it is not limited by them, since it cannot only give them new directions and much variation, refining and extension, but is able to act in thought and imagination and a mental world of much more subtle and flexible creations. But also there is an intuition in the mental Purusha of something larger and greater than this present action in which he lives, a range of experience of which it is only a frontal scheme or a narrow superficial selection. By this intuition he stands upon the threshold of a subliminal self with a more extended possibility than this superficial mentality opens to his self-knowledge. A last and greatest intuition is an inner awareness of something which he more essentially is, something as high above mind as mind is above the physical life and body. This inner awareness is his intuition of his supramental and spiritual being.

The mental Purusha can at any time involve himself again in the superficial action from which he has drawn back, live for a while entirely identified with the mechanism of mind, life and body and absorbedly repeat its recurrent normal action. But once that separative movement has been made and lived in for some time, he can never be to himself quite what he was before. The involution in the outward action becomes now only a recurrent self-oblivion from which there is a tendency in him to draw back again to himself and to pure self-experience. It may be noted too that the Purusha by drawing back from the normal action of this outward consciousness which has created for him his present natural form of self-experience, is able to take two other poises. He can have an intuition of himself as a soul in body, which puts forth life as its activity and mind as the light of that activity. This soul in body is the physical conscious being, *annamaya puruṣa*, which uses life and mind characteristically for physical experience,—all else being regarded as a consequence of physical experience,—does not look beyond the life of the body and, so far as it feels anything beyond its physical individuality, is aware only of the physical universe and at most its oneness with the soul of physical Nature. But he can have too an intuition of himself as a soul of life, self-identified with a great movement of becoming in Time, which puts forth body as a form or basic sense-image and mind as a conscious activity of life-experience. This soul in life is the vital conscious being, *prāṇamaya puruṣa*, which is capable of looking beyond the duration and limits of the physical body, of feeling an eternity of life behind and in front, an identity with a universal Life-being, but does not look beyond a constant vital becoming in Time. These three Purushas are soul-forms of the Spirit by which it identifies its conscious existence with and founds its action upon any of these three planes or principles of its universal being.

But man is characteristically a mental being. Moreover, mentality is his highest present status in which he is nearest to his real self, most easily and largely aware of spirit. His way to perfection is not to involve himself in the outward or superficial existence, nor is it to place himself in the soul of life or the soul of body, but to insist on the three mental intuitions by which he can lift himself eventually above the physical, vital and mental levels. This insistence may take two quite different forms, each with its own object and way of proceeding. It is quite possible for him to accentuate it in a direction away from existence in Nature, a detachment, a withdrawal from mind, life and body. He may try to live more and more as the witness Purusha, regarding the action of Nature, without interest in it, without sanction to it, detached, rejecting the whole action, withdrawing into pure conscious existence. This is the Sankhya liberation. He may go inward into that larger existence of which he has the intuition and away from the superficial mentality into a dream-state or sleep-state which admits him into wider or higher ranges of consciousness. By passing away into these ranges he may put away from him the terrestrial being. There is even, it was supposed in ancient times, a transition to supramental worlds from which a return to earthly consciousness was either not possible or not obligatory. But the definite and sure finality of this kind of liberation depends on the elevation of the mental being into that spiritual self of which he becomes aware when he looks away and upward from all mentality. That is given as the key to entire cessation from terrestrial existence whether by immergence in pure being or a participation in supracosmic being.

But if our aim is to be not only free by self-detachment from Nature, but perfected in mastery, this type of insistence can no longer suffice. We have to regard our mental, vital and physical action of Nature, find out the knots of its bondage and the loosing-points of liberation, discover the keys of its imperfection and lay our finger on the key of perfection. When the regarding soul, the witness Purusha stands back from his action of nature and observes it, he sees that it proceeds of its own impulsion by the power of its mechanism, by force of continuity of movement, continuity of mentality, continuity of life impulse, continuity of an involuntary physical mechanism. At first the whole thing seems to be the recurrent action of an automatic machinery, although the sum of that action mounts constantly into a creation, development, evolution. He was as if seized in this wheel, attached to it by the ego sense, whirled round and onward in the circling of the machinery. A complete mechanical determinism or a stream of determinations of Nature to which he lent the light of his consciousness, is the natural aspect of his mental, vital and physical personality once it is regarded from this stable detached standpoint and no longer by a soul caught up in the movement and imagining itself to be a part of the action.

But on a farther view we find that this determinism is not so complete as it seemed; action of Nature continues and is what it is because of the sanction of the Purusha. The regarding Purusha sees that he supports and in some way fills and pervades the action with his conscious being. He discovers that without him it could not continue and that where he persistently withdraws this sanction, the habitual action becomes gradually enfeebled, flags and ceases. His whole active mentality can be thus brought to a complete stillness. There is yet a passive mentality which mechanically continues, but this too can be stilled by his withdrawal into himself out of the action. Even then the life action in its most mechanical parts continues; but that too can be stilled into cessation. It would appear then that he is not only the upholding (*bhartṛ*) Purusha, but in some way the master of his nature, Ishwara. It was the consciousness of this sanctioning control, this necessity of his consent, which made him in the ego-sense conceive of himself as a soul or mental being with a free will determining all his own becomings. Yet the free-will seems to be imperfect, almost illusory, since the actual will itself is a machinery of Nature and each separate willing determined by the stream of past action and the sum of conditions it created,— although, because the result of the stream, the sum, is at each moment a new development, a new determination, it may seem to be a self-born willing, virginally creative at each moment. What he contributed all the while was a consent behind, a sanction to what Nature was doing. He does not seem able to rule her entirely, but only choose between certain well-defined possibilities: there is in her a power of resistance born of her past impetus and a still greater power of resistance born of the sum of fixed conditions she has created, which she presents to him as a set of permanent laws to be obeyed. He cannot radically alter her way of proceeding, cannot freely effect his will from within her present movement, nor, while standing in the mentality, get outside or above her in such a way as to exercise a really free control. There is a duality of dependence, her dependence on his consent, his dependence on her law and way and limits of action, determination denied by a sense of free-will, free-will nullified by the actuality of natural determination. He is sure that she is his power, but yet he seems to be subject to her. He is the sanctioning (*anumantṛ*) Purusha, but does not seem to be the absolute lord, Ishwara.

Nevertheless, there is somewhere an absolute control, a real Ishwara.

He is aware of it and knows that if he can find it, he will enter into control, become not only the passive sanctioning witness and upholding soul of her will, but the free powerful user and determiner of her movements. But this control seems to belong to another poise than the mentality. Sometimes he finds himself using it, but as a channel or instrument; it comes to him from above. It is clear then that it is supramental, a power of the Spirit greater than mental being which he already knows himself to be at the summit and in the secret core of his conscious being. To enter into identity with that Spirit must then be his way to control and lordship. He can do it passively by a sort of reflection and receiving in his mental consciousness, but then he is only a mould, channel or instrument, not a possessor or participant in the power. He can arrive at identity by an absorption of his mentality in inner spiritual being, but then the conscious action ceases in a trance of identity. To be active master of the nature he must evidently rise to some higher supramental poise where there is possible not only a passive, but an active identity with the controlling spirit. To find the way of rising to this greater poise and be self-ruler, Swarat, is a condition of his perfection.

The difficulty of the ascent is due to a natural ignorance. He is the Purusha, witness of mental and physical Nature, *sākṣī*, but not a complete knower of self and Nature, *jñātṛ*. Knowledge in the mentality is enlightened by his consciousness; he is the mental knower; but he finds that this is not a real knowledge, but only a partial seeking and partial finding, a derivative uncertain reflection and narrow utilisation for action from a greater light beyond which is the real knowledge. This light is the self-awareness and all-awareness of Spirit. The essential self-awareness he can arrive at even on the mental plane of being, by reflection in the soul of mind or by its absorption in spirit, as indeed it can be arrived at by another kind of reflection or absorption in soul of life and soul of body. But for participation in an effective all-awareness with this essential self-awareness as the soul of its action he must rise to supermind. To be lord of his being, he must be knower of self and Nature, *jñātā īśvaraḥ*. Partially this may be done on a higher level of mind where it responds directly to supermind, but really and completely this perfection belongs not to the mental being, but to the ideal or knowledge Soul, *vijñānamaya puruṣa*. To draw up the mental into the greater knowledge being and that into the Bliss-Self of the spirit, *ānandamaya puruṣa*, is the uttermost way of this perfection.

But no perfection, much less this perfection can be attained without a very radical dealing with the present nature and the abrogation of much that seems to be the fixed law of its complex nexus of mental, vital and physical being. The law of this nexus has been created for a definite and limited end, the temporary maintenance, preservation, possession, aggrandisement, enjoyment, experience, need, action of the mental ego in the living body. Other resultant uses are served, but this is the immediate and fundamentally determining object and utility. To arrive at a higher utility and freer instrumentation this nexus must be partly broken up, exceeded, transformed into a larger harmony of action. The Purusha sees that the law created is that of a partly stable, partly unstable selective determination of habitual, yet developing experiences out of a first confused consciousness of self and not-self, subjective being and external universe. This determination is managed by mind, life and body acting upon each other, in harmony and correspondence, but also in discord and divergence, mutual interference and limitation. There is a similar mixed harmony and discord between various activities of the mind in itself, as also between activities of the life in itself and of the physical being. The whole is a sort of disorderly order, an order evolved and contrived out of a constantly surrounding and invading confusion.

This is the first difficulty the Purusha has to deal with, a mixed and confused action of Nature,—an action without clear self-knowledge, distinct motive, firm instrumentation, only an attempt at these things and a general relative success of effectuality,—a surprising effect of adaptation in some directions, but also much distress of inadequacy. That mixed and confused action has to be mended; purification is an essential means towards self-perfection. All these impurities and inadequacies result in various kinds of limitation and bondage: but there are two or three primary knots of the bondage,—ego is the principal knot,—from which the others derive. These bonds must be got rid of; purification is not complete till it brings about liberation. Besides, after a certain purification and liberation has been effected, there is still the conversion of the purified instruments to the law of a higher object and utility, a large, real and perfect order of action. By the conversion man can arrive at a certain perfection of fullness of being, calm, power and knowledge, even a greater vital action and more perfect physical existence. One result of this perfection is a large and perfected delight of being, Ananda. Thus purification, liberation, perfection, delight of being are four constituent elements of the Yoga,—*śuddhi, mukti, siddhi, bhukti.*

But this perfection cannot be attained or cannot be secure and entire in its largeness if the Purusha lays stress on individuality. To abandon identification with the physical, vital and mental ego, is not enough; he must arrive in soul also at a true, universalised, not separative individuality. In the lower nature man is an ego making a clean cut in conception between himself and all other existence; the ego is to him self, but all the rest not self, external to his being. His whole action starts from and is founded upon this self-conception and world-conception. But the conception is in fact an error. However sharply he individualises himself in mental idea and mental or other action, he is inseparable from the universal being, his body from universal force and matter, his life from the universal life, his mind from universal mind, his soul and spirit from universal soul and spirit. The universal acts on him, invades him, overcomes him, shapes itself in him at every moment; he in his reaction acts on the universal, invades, tries to impose himself on it, shape it, overcome its attack, rule and use its instrumentation.

This conflict is a rendering of the underlying unity, which assumes the aspect of struggle by a necessity of the original separation; the two pieces into which mind has cut the oneness, rush upon each other to restore the oneness and each tries to seize on and take into itself the separated portion. Universe seems to be always trying to swallow up man, the infinite to resume this finite which stands on its self-defence and even replies by aggression. But in real fact the universal being through this apparent struggle is working out its purpose in man, though the key and truth of the purpose and working is lost to his superficial conscious mind, only held obscurely in an underlying subconscient and only known luminously in an overruling superconscient unity. Man also is impelled towards unity by a constant impulse of extension of his ego, which identifies itself as best it can with other egos and with such portions of the universe as he can physically, vitally, mentally get into his use and possession. As man aims at knowledge and mastery of his own being, so also he aims at knowledge and mastery of the environmental world of nature, its objects, its instrumentation, its beings. First he tries to effect this aim by egoistic possession, but, as he develops, the element of sympathy born of the secret oneness grows in him and he arrives at the idea of a widening cooperation and oneness with other beings, a harmony with universal Nature and universal being.

The witness Purusha in the mind observes that the inadequacy of his effort, all the inadequacy in fact of man's life and nature arises from the separation and the consequent struggle, want of knowledge, want of harmony, want of oneness. It is essential for him to grow out of separative individuality, to universalise himself, to make himself one with the universe. This unification can be done only through the soul by making our soul of mind one with the universal Mind, our soul of life one with the universal Life-soul, our soul of body one with the universal soul of physical Nature. When this can be done, in proportion to the power, intensity, depth, completeness, permanence with which it can be done, great effects are produced upon the natural action. Especially there grows an immediate and profound sympathy and immixture of mind with mind, life with life, a lessening of the body's insistence on separateness, a power of direct mental and other intercommunication and effective mutual action which helps out now the inadequate indirect communication and action that was till now the greater part of the conscious means used by embodied mind. But still the Purusha sees that in mental, vital, physical nature, taken by itself, there is always a defect, inadequacy, confused action, due to the mechanically unequal interplay of the three modes or gunas of Nature. To transcend it he has in the universality too to rise to the supramental and spiritual, to be one with the supramental soul of cosmos, the universal spirit. He arrives at the larger light and order of a higher principle in himself and the universe which is the characteristic action of the divine Sachchidananda. Even, he is able to impose the influence of that light and order, not only on his own natural being, but, within the radius and to the extent of the Spirit's action in him, on the world he lives in, on that which is around him. He is *svarāṭ*, self-knower, self-ruler, but he begins to be also through this spiritual oneness and transcendence *samrāṭ*, a knower and master of his environing world of being.

In this self-development the soul finds that it has accomplished on this line the object of the whole integral Yoga, union with the Supreme in its self and in its universalised individuality. So long as he remains in the world-existence, this perfection must radiate out from him,—for that is the necessity of his oneness with the universe and its beings,—in an influence and action which help all around who are capable of it to rise to or advance towards the same perfection, and for the rest in an influence and action which help, as only the self-ruler and master man can help, in leading the human race forward spiritually towards this consummation and towards some image of a greater divine truth in their personal and communal existence. He becomes a light and power of the Truth to which he has climbed and a means for others' ascension.

# THE INSTRUMENTS OF THE SPIRIT

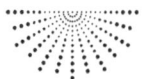

IF THERE is to be an active perfection of our being, the first necessity is a purification of the working of the instruments which it now uses for a music of discords. The being itself, the spirit, the divine Reality in man stands in no need of purification; it is for ever pure, not affected by the faults of its instrumentation or the stumblings of mind and heart and body in their work, as the sun, says the Upanishad, is not touched or stained by the faults of the eye of vision. Mind, heart, the soul of vital desire, the life in the body are the seats of impurity; it is they that must be set right if the working of the spirit is to be a perfect working and not marked by its present greater or less concession to the devious pleasure of the lower nature. What is ordinarily called purity of the being, is either a negative whiteness, a freedom from sin gained by a constant inhibition of whatever action, feeling, idea or will we think to be wrong, or else, the highest negative or passive purity, the entire God-content, inaction, the complete stilling of the vibrant mind and the soul of desire, which in quietistic disciplines leads to a supreme peace; for then the spirit appears in all the eternal purity of its immaculate essence. That gained, there would be nothing farther to be enjoyed or done. But here we have the more difficult problem of a total, unabated, even an increased and more powerful action founded on perfect bliss of the being, the purity of the soul's instrumental as well as the spirit's essential nature. Mind, heart, life, body are to do the works of the Divine, all the works which they do now and yet more, but to do them divinely, as now they do not do them. This is the first appearance of the problem before him on which the seeker of perfection has to lay hold, that it is not a negative, prohibitory, passive or quietistic, but a positive, affirmative, active purity which is his object. A divine quietism discovers the immaculate eternity of the Spirit, a divine kinetism adds to it the right pure undeviating action of the soul, mind and body.

Moreover, it is a total purification of all the complex instrumentality in all the parts of each instrument that is demanded of us by the integral perfection. It is not, ultimately, the narrower moral purification of the ethical nature. Ethics deals only with the desire-soul and the active outward dynamical part of our being; its field is confined to character and action. It prohibits and inhibits certain actions, certain desires, impulses, propensities,—it inculcates certain qualities in the act, such as truthfulness, love, charity, compassion, chastity. When it has got this done and assured a base of virtue, the possession of a purified will and blameless habit of action, its work is finished. But the Siddha of the integral perfection has to dwell in a larger plane of the Spirit's eternal purity beyond good and evil. By this phrase it is not meant, as the rash hastily concluding intellect would be prone to imagine, that he will do good and evil indifferently and declare that to the spirit there is no difference between them, which would be in the plane of individual action an obvious untruth and might serve to cover a reckless self-indulgence of the imperfect human nature. Neither is it meant that since good and evil are in this world inextricably entangled together, like pain and pleasure, —a proposition which, however true at the moment and plausible as a generalisation, need not be true of the human being's greater spiritual evolution,—the liberated man will live in the spirit and stand back from the mechanical continued workings of a necessarily imperfect nature. This, however possible as a stage towards a final cessation of all activity, is evidently not a counsel of active perfection. But it is meant that the Siddha of the active integral perfection will live dynamically in the working of the transcendent power of the divine Spirit as a universal will through the supermind individualised in him for action. His works will therefore be the works of an eternal Knowledge, an eternal Truth, an eternal Might, an eternal Love, an eternal Ananda; but the truth, knowledge, force, love, delight will be the whole essential spirit of whatever work he will do and will not depend on its form; they will determine his action from the spirit within and the action will not determine the spirit or subject it to a fixed standard or rigid mould of working. He will have no dominant mere habit of character, but only a spiritual being and will with at the most a free and flexible temperamental mould for the action. His life will be a direct stream from the eternal fountains, not a form cut to some temporary human pattern. His perfection will not be a sattwic purity, but a thing uplifted beyond the gunas of Nature, a perfection of spiritual knowledge, spiritual power, spiritual delight, unity and harmony of unity; the outward perfection of his works will be freely shaped as the self-expression of this inner spiritual transcendence and universality. For this change he must make conscient in him that power of spirit and supermind which is now superconscient to our mentality. But that cannot work in him so long as his present mental, vital, physical being is not liberated from its actual inferior working. This purification is the first necessity.

In other words, purification must not be understood in any limited sense of a selection of certain outward kinetic movements, their regulation, the inhibition of other action or a liberation of certain forms of character or particular mental and moral capacities. These things are secondary signs of our derivative being, not essential powers and first forces. We have to take a wider psychological view of the primary forces of our nature. We have to distinguish the formed parts of our being, find out their basic defect of impurity or wrong action and correct that, sure that the rest will then come right naturally. We have not to doctor symptoms of impurity, or that only secondarily, as a minor help,—but to strike at its roots after a deeper diagnosis. We then find that there are two forms of impurity which are at the root of the whole confusion. One is a defect born of the nature of our past evolution, which has been a nature of separative ignorance; this defect is a radically wrong and ignorant form given to the proper action of each part of our instrumental being. The other impurity is born of the successive process of an evolution, where life emerges in and depends on body, mind emerges in and depends on life in the body, supermind emerges in and lends itself to instead of governing mind, soul itself is apparent only as a circumstance of the bodily life of the mental being and veils up the spirit in the lower imperfections. This second defect of our nature is caused by this dependence of the higher on the lower parts; it is an immixture of functions by which the impure working of the lower instrument gets into the characteristic action of the higher function and gives to it an added imperfection of embarrassment, wrong direction and confusion.

Thus the proper function of the life, the vital force, is enjoyment and possession, both of them perfectly legitimate, because the Spirit created the world for Ananda, enjoyment and possession of the many by the One, of the One by the many and of the many too by the many; but,—this is an instance of the first kind of defect,—the separative ignorance gives to it the wrong form of desire and craving which vitiates the whole enjoyment and possession and imposes on it its opposites, want and suffering. Again, because mind is entangled in life from which it evolves, this desire and craving get into the action of the mental will and knowledge; that makes the will a will of craving, a force of desire instead of a rational will and a discerning force of intelligent effectuation, and it distorts the judgment and reason so that we judge and reason according to our desires and prepossessions and not with the disinterested impartiality of a pure judgment and the rectitude of a reason which seeks only to distinguish truth and understand rightly the objects of its workings. That is an example of immixture. These two kinds of defect, wrong form of action and illegitimate mixture of action, are not limited to these signal instances, but belong to each instrument and to each combination of their functionings. They pervade the whole economy of our nature. They are fundamental defects of our lower instrumental nature, and if we can set them right, we shall get our instrumental being into a state of purity, enjoy the clarity of a pure will, a pure heart of emotion, a pure enjoyment of our vitality, a pure body. That will be a preliminary, a human perfection, but it can be made the basis and open out in its effort of self-attainment into the greater, the divine perfection.

Mind, life and body are the three powers of our lower nature. But they cannot be taken quite separately because the life acts as a link and gives its character to body and to a great extent to our mentality. Our body is a living body; the life-force mingles in and determines all its functionings. Our mind too is largely a mind of life, a mind of physical sensation; only in its higher functions is it normally capable of something more than the workings of a physical mentality subjected to life. We may put it in this ascending order. We have first a body supported by the physical life-force, the physical prana which courses through the whole nervous system and gives its stamp to our corporeal action, so that all is of the character of the action of a living and not an inert mechanical body. Prana and physicality together make the gross body, *sthūla śarīra*. This is only the outer instrument, the nervous force of life acting in the form of body with its gross physical organs. Then there is the inner instrument, *antaḥkaraṇa*, the conscious mentality. This inner instrument is divided by the old system into four powers; *citta* or basic mental consciousness; *manas*, the sense mind; *buddhi*, the intelligence; *ahaṅkāra*, the ego-idea. The classification may serve as a starting-point, though for a greater practicality we have to make certain farther distinctions. This mentality is pervaded by the life-force, which becomes here an instrument for psychic consciousness of life and psychic action on life. Every fibre of the sense mind and basic consciousness is shot through with the action of this psychic prana, it is a nervous or vital and physical mentality. Even the buddhi and ego are overpowered by it, although they have the capacity of raising the mind beyond subjection to this vital, nervous and physical psychology. This combination creates in us the sensational desire-soul which is the chief obstacle to a higher human as well as to the still greater divine perfection. Finally, above our present conscious mentality is a secret supermind which is the proper means and native seat of that perfection.

Chitta, the basic consciousness, is largely subconscient; it has, open and hidden, two kinds of action, one passive or receptive, the other active or reactive and formative. As a passive power it receives all impacts, even those of which the mind is unaware or to which it is inattentive, and it stores them in an immense reserve of passive subconscient memory on which the mind as an active memory can draw. But ordinarily the mind draws only what it had observed and understood at the time,—more easily what it had observed well and understood carefully, less easily what it had observed carelessly or ill understood; at the same time there is a power in consciousness to send up to the active mind for use what that mind had not at all observed or attended to or even consciously experienced. This power only acts observably in abnormal conditions, when some part of the subconscious chitta comes as it were to the surface or when the subliminal being in us appears on the threshold and for a time plays some part in the outer chamber of mentality where the direct intercourse and commerce with the external world takes place and our inner dealings with ourselves develop on the surface. This action of memory is so fundamental to the entire mental action that it is sometimes said, memory is the man. Even in the submental action of the body and life, which is full of this subconscient chitta, though not under the control of the conscious mind, there is a vital and physical memory. The vital and physical habits are largely formed by this submental memory. For this reason they can be changed to an indefinite extent by a more powerful action of conscious mind and will, when that can be developed and can find means to communicate to the subconscient chitta the will of the spirit for a new law of vital and physical action. Even, the whole constitution of our life and body may be described as a bundle of habits formed by the past evolution in Nature and held together by the persistent memory of this secret consciousness. For chitta, the primary stuff of consciousness, is like prana and body universal in Nature, but is subconscient and mechanical in nature of Matter.

But in fact all action of the mind or inner instrument arises out of this chitta or basic consciousness, partly conscient, partly subconscient or subliminal to our active mentality. When it is struck by the world's impacts from outside or urged by the reflective powers of the subjective inner being, it throws up certain habitual activities, the mould of which has been determined by our evolution. One of these forms of activity is the emotional mind,—the heart, as we may call it for the sake of a convenient brevity. Our emotions are the waves of reaction and response which rise up from the basic consciousness, *citta-vṛtti*. Their action too is largely regulated by habit and an emotive memory. They are not imperative, not laws of Necessity; there is no really binding law of our emotional being to which we must submit without remedy; we are not obliged to give responses of grief to certain impacts upon the mind, responses of anger to others, to yet others responses of hatred or dislike, to others responses of liking or love. All these things are only habits of our affective mentality; they can be changed by the conscious will of the spirit; they can be inhibited; we may even rise entirely above all subjection to grief, anger, hatred, the duality of liking and disliking. We are subject to these things only so long as we persist in subjection to the mechanical action of the chitta in the emotive mentality, a thing difficult to get rid of because of the power of past habit and especially the importunate insistence of the vital part of mentality, the nervous life-mind or psychic prana. This nature of the emotive mind as a reaction of chitta with a certain close dependence upon the nervous life sensations and the responses of the psychic prana is so characteristic that in some languages it is called chitta and prana, the heart, the life soul; it is indeed the most directly agitating and powerfully insistent action of the desire-soul which the immixture of vital desire and responsive consciousness has created in us. And yet the true emotive soul, the real psyche in us, is not a desire-soul, but a soul of pure love and delight; but that, like the rest of our true being, can only emerge when the deformation created by the life of desire is removed from the surface and is no longer the characteristic action of our being. To get that done is a necessary part of our purification, liberation, perfection.

The nervous action of the psychic prana is most obvious in our purely sensational mentality. This nervous mentality pursues indeed all the action of the inner instrument and seems often to form the greater part of things other than sensation. The emotions are especially assailed and have the pranic stamp; fear is more even of a nervous sensation than an emotion, anger is largely or often a sensational response translated into terms of emotion. Other feelings are more of the heart, more inward, but they ally themselves to the nervous and physical longings or outward-going impulses of the psychic prana. Love is an emotion of the heart and may be a pure feeling,—all mentality, since we are embodied minds, must produce, even thought produces, some kind of life effect and some response in the stuff of body, but they need not for that reason be of a physical nature,—but the heart's love allies itself readily with a vital desire in the body. This physical element may be purified of that subjection to physical desire which is called lust, it may become love using the body for a physical as well as a mental and spiritual nearness; but love may, too, separate itself from all, even the most innocent physical element, or from all but a shadow of it, and be a pure movement to union of soul with soul, psyche with psyche. Still the proper action of the sensational mind is not emotion, but conscious nervous response and nervous feeling and affection, impulse of the use of physical sense and body for some action, conscious vital craving and desire. There is a side of receptive response, a side of dynamic reaction. These things get their proper normal use when the higher mind is not mechanically subject to them, but controls and regulates their action. But a still higher state is when they undergo a certain transformation by the conscious will of the spirit which gives its right and no longer its wrong or desire form of characteristic action to the psychic prana.

Manas, the sense mind, depends in our ordinary consciousness on the physical organs of receptive sense for knowledge and on the organs of the body for action directed towards the objects of sense. The superficial and outward action of the senses is physical and nervous in its character, and they may easily be thought to be merely results of nerve-action; they are sometimes called in the old books *prāṇas*, nervous or life activities. But still the essential thing in them is not the nervous excitation, but the consciousness, the action of the chitta, which makes use of the organ and of the nervous impact of which it is the channel. Manas, sense-mind, is the activity, emerging from the basic consciousness, which makes up the whole essentiality of what we call sense. Sight, hearing, taste, smell, touch are really properties of the mind, not of the body; but the physical mind which we ordinarily use, limits itself to a translation into sense of so much of the outer impacts as it receives through the nervous system and the physical organs. But the inner Manas has also a subtle sight, hearing, power of contact of its own which is not dependent on the physical organs. And it has, moreover, a power not only of direct communication of mind with object—leading even at a high pitch of action to a sense of the contents of an object within or beyond the physical range,—but direct communication also of mind with mind. Mind is able too to alter, modify, inhibit the incidence, values, intensities of sense impacts. These powers of the mind we do not ordinarily use or develop; they remain subliminal and emerge sometimes in an irregular and fitful action, more readily in some minds than in others, or come to the surface in abnormal states of the being. They are the basis of clairvoyance, clairaudience, transference of thought and impulse, telepathy, most of the more ordinary kinds of occult powers,—so called, though these are better described less mystically as powers of the now subliminal action of the Manas. The phenomena of hypnotism and many others depend upon the action of this subliminal sense-mind; not that it alone constitutes all the elements of the phenomena, but it is the first supporting means of intercourse, communication and response, though much of the actual operation belongs to an inner Buddhi. Mind physical, mind supraphysical,—we have and can use this double sense mentality.

Buddhi is a construction of conscious being which quite exceeds its beginnings in the basic chitta; it is the intelligence with its power of knowledge and will. Buddhi takes up and deals with all the rest of the action of the mind and life and body. It is in its nature thought-power and will-power of the Spirit turned into the lower form of a mental activity. We may distinguish three successive gradations of the action of this intelligence. There is first an inferior perceptive understanding which simply takes up, records, understands and responds to the communications of the sense-mind, memory, heart and sensational mentality. It creates by their means an elementary thinking mind which does not go beyond their data, but subjects itself to their mould and rings out their repetitions, runs round and round in the habitual circle of thought and will suggested by them or follows, with an obedient subservience of the reason to the suggestions of life, any fresh determinations which may be offered to its perception and conception. Beyond this elementary understanding, which we all use to an enormous extent, there is a power of arranging or selecting reason and will-force of the intelligence which has for its action and aim an attempt to arrive at a plausible, sufficient, settled ordering of knowledge and will for the use of an intellectual conception of life.

In spite of its more purely intellectual character this secondary or intermediate reason is really pragmatic in its intention. It creates a certain kind of intellectual structure, frame, rule into which it tries to cast the inner and outer life so as to use it with a certain mastery and government for the purposes of some kind of rational will. It is this reason which gives to our normal intellectual being our set aesthetic and ethical standards, our structures of opinion and our established norms of idea and purpose. It is highly developed and takes the primacy in all men of an at all developed understanding. But beyond it there is a reason, a highest action of the buddhi which concerns itself disinterestedly with a pursuit of pure truth and right knowledge; it seeks to discover the real Truth behind life and things and our apparent selves and to subject its will to the law of Truth. Few, if any of us, can use this highest reason with any purity, but the attempt to do it is the topmost capacity of the inner instrument, the *antaḥkaraṇa*.

Buddhi is really an intermediary between a much higher Truth-mind not now in our active possession, which is the direct instrument of Spirit, and the physical life of the human mind evolved in body. Its powers of intelligence and will are drawn from this greater direct Truth-mind or supermind. Buddhi centres its mental action round the ego-idea, the idea that I am this mind, life and body or am a mental being determined by their action. It serves this ego-idea whether limited by what we call egoism or extended by sympathy with the life around us. An ego-sense is created which reposes on the separative action of the body, of the individualised life, of the mind-responses, and the ego-idea in the buddhi centralises the whole action of this ego's thought, character, personality. The lower understanding and the intermediary reason are instruments of its desire of experience and self-enlargement. But when the highest reason and will develop, we can turn towards that which these outward things mean to the higher spiritual consciousness. The "I" can then be seen as a mental reflection of the Self, the Spirit, the Divine, the one existence transcendent, universal, individual in its multiplicity; the consciousness in which these things meet, become aspects of one being and assume their right relations, can then be unveiled out of all these physical and mental coverings. When the transition to supermind takes place, the powers of the Buddhi do not perish, but have all to be converted to their supramental values. But the consideration of the supermind and the conversion of the buddhi belongs to the question of the higher siddhi or divine perfection. At present we have to consider the purification of the normal being of man, preparatory to any such conversion, which leads to the liberation from the bonds of our lower nature.

# PURIFICATION — THE LOWER MENTALITY

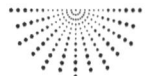

WE HAVE to deal with the complex action of all these instruments and set about their purification. And the simplest way will be to fasten on the two kinds of radical defect in each, distinguish clearly in what they consist and set them right. But there is also the question where we are to begin. For the entanglement is great, the complete purification of one instrument depends on the complete purification too of all the others, and that is a great source of difficulty, disappointment and perplexity,—as when we think we have got the intelligence purified, only to find that it is still subject to attack and overclouding because the emotions of the heart and the will and sensational mind are still affected by the many impurities of the lower nature and they get back into the enlightened buddhi and prevent it from reflecting the pure truth for which we are seeking. But we have on the other hand this advantage that one important instrument sufficiently purified can be used as a means for the purification of the others, one step firmly taken makes easier all the others and gets rid of a host of difficulties. Which instrument then by its purification and perfection will bring about most easily and effectively or can aid with a most powerful rapidity the perfection of the rest?

Since we are the spirit enveloped in mind, a soul evolved here as a mental being in a living physical body, it must naturally be in the mind, the *antaḥkaraṇa*, that we must look for this desideratum. And in the mind it is evidently by the buddhi, the intelligence and the will of the intelligence that the human being is intended to do whatever work is not done for him by the physical or nervous nature as in the plant and the animal. Pending the evolution of any higher supramental power the intelligent will must be our main force for effectuation and to purify it becomes a very primary necessity. Once our intelligence and will are well purified of all that limits them and gives them a wrong action or wrong direction, they can easily be perfected, can be made to respond to the suggestions of Truth, understand themselves and the rest of the being, see clearly and with a fine and scrupulous accuracy what they are doing and follow out the right way to do it without any hesitating or eager error or stumbling deviation. Eventually their response can be opened up to the perfect discernings, intuitions, inspirations, revelations of the supermind and proceed by a more and more luminous and even infallible action. But this purification cannot be effected without a preliminary clearing of its natural obstacles in the other lower parts of the *antaḥkaraṇa*, and the chief natural obstacle running through the whole action of the *antaḥkaraṇa*, through the sense, the mental sensation, emotion, dynamic impulse, intelligence, will, is the intermiscence and the compelling claim of the psychic prana. This then must be dealt with, its dominating intermiscence ruled out, its claim denied, itself quieted and prepared for purification.

Each instrument has, it has been said, a proper and legitimate action and also a deformation or wrong principle of its proper action. The proper action of the psychic prana is pure possession and enjoyment, *bhoga*. To enjoy thought, will, action, dynamic impulse, result of action, emotion, sense, sensation, to enjoy too by their means objects, persons, life, the world, is the activity for which this prana gives us a psycho-physical basis. A really perfect enjoyment of existence can only come when what we enjoy is not the world in itself or for itself, but God in the world, when it is not things, but the Ananda of the spirit in things that forms the real, essential object of our enjoying and things only as form and symbol of the spirit, waves of the ocean of Ananda. But this Ananda can only come at all when we can get at and reflect in our members the hidden spiritual being, and its fullness can only be had when we climb to the supramental ranges. Meanwhile there is a just and permissible, a quite legitimate human enjoyment of these things, which is, to speak in the language of Indian psychology, predominantly sattwic in its nature. It is an enlightened enjoyment principally by the perceptive, aesthetic and emotive mind, secondarily only by the sensational, nervous and physical being, but all subject to the clear government of the buddhi, to a right reason, a right will, a right reception of the life impacts, a right order, a right feeling of the truth, law, ideal sense, beauty, use of things. The mind gets the pure taste of enjoyment of them, *rasa*, and rejects whatever is perturbed, troubled and perverse. Into this acceptance of the clear and limpid *rasa*, the psychic prana has to bring in the full sense of life and the occupying enjoyment by the whole being, *bhoga*, without which the acceptance and possession by the mind, *rasa-grahaṇa*, would not be concrete enough, would be too tenuous to satisfy altogether the embodied soul. This contribution is its proper function.

The deformation which enters in and prevents the purity, is a form of vital craving; the grand deformation which the psychic prana contributes to our being, is desire. The root of desire is the vital craving to seize upon that which we feel we have not, it is the limited life's instinct for possession and satisfaction. It creates the sense of want,—first the simpler vital craving of hunger, thirst, lust, then these psychical hungers, thirsts, lusts of the mind which are a much greater and more instant and pervading affliction of our being, the hunger which is infinite because it is the hunger of an infinite being, the thirst which is only temporarily lulled by satisfaction, but is in its nature insatiable. The psychic prana invades the sensational mind and brings into it the unquiet thirst of sensations, invades the dynamic mind with the lust of control, having, domination, success, fulfilment of every impulse, fills the emotional mind with the desire for the satisfaction of liking and disliking, for the wreaking of love and hate, brings the shrinkings and panics of fear and the strainings and disappointments of hope, imposes the tortures of grief and the brief fevers and excitements of joy, makes the intelligence and intelligent will the accomplices of all these things and turns them in their own kind into deformed and lame instruments, the will into a will of craving and the intelligence into a partial, a stumbling and an eager pursuer of limited, impatient, militant prejudgment and opinion. Desire is the root of all sorrow, disappointment, affliction, for though it has a feverish joy of pursuit and satisfaction, yet because it is always a straining of the being, it carries into its pursuit and its getting a labour, hunger, struggle, a rapid subjection to fatigue, a sense of limitation, dissatisfaction and early disappointment with all its gains, a ceaseless morbid stimulation, trouble, disquiet, *aśānti*. To get rid of desire is the one firm indispensable purification of the psychical prana,—for so we can replace the soul of desire with its pervading immiscence in all our instruments by a mental soul of calm delight and its clear and limpid possession of ourselves and world and Nature which is the crystal basis of the mental life and its perfection.

The psychical prana interferes in all the higher operations to deform them, but its defect is itself due to its being interfered with and deformed by the nature of the physical workings in the body which Life has evolved in its emergence from matter. It is that which has created the separation of the individual life in the body from the life of the universe and stamped on it the character of want, limitation, hunger, thirst, craving for what it has not, a long groping after enjoyment and a hampered and baffled need of possession. Easily regulated and limited in the purely physical order of things, it extends itself in the psychical prana immensely and becomes, as the mind grows, a thing with difficulty limited, insatiable, irregular, a busy creator of disorder and disease. Moreover, the psychical prana leans on the physical life, limits itself by the nervous force of the physical being, limits thereby the operations of the mind and becomes the link of its dependence on the body and its subjection to fatigue, incapacity, disease, disorder, insanity, the pettiness, the precariousness and even the possible dissolution of the workings of the physical mentality. Our mind instead of being a thing powerful in its own strength, a clear instrument of conscious spirit, free and able to control, use and perfect the life and body, appears in the result a mixed construction; it is a predominantly physical mentality limited by its physical organs and subject to the demands and to the obstructions of the life in the body. This can only be got rid of by a sort of practical, inward psychological operation of analysis by which we become aware of the mentality as a separate power, isolate it for a free working, distinguish too the psychical and the physical prana and make them no longer a link for dependence, but a transmitting channel for the Idea and Will in the buddhi, obedient to its suggestions and commands; the prana then becomes a passive means of effectuation for the mind's direct control of the physical life. This control, however abnormal to our habitual poise of action, is not only possible,—it appears to some extent in the phenomena of hypnosis, though these are unhealthily abnormal, because there it is a foreign will which suggests and commands,—but must become the normal action when the higher Self within takes up the direct command of the whole being. This control can be exercised perfectly, however, only from the supramental level, for it is there that the true effective Idea and

Will reside and the mental thought-mind, even spiritualised, is only a limited, though it may be made a very powerful deputy.

Desire, it is thought, is the real motive power of human living and to cast it out would be to stop the springs of life; satisfaction of desire is man's only enjoyment and to eliminate it would be to extinguish the impulse of life by a quietistic asceticism. But the real motive power of the life of the soul is Will; desire is only a deformation of will in the dominant bodily life and physical mind. The essential turn of the soul to possession and enjoyment of the world consists in a will to delight, and the enjoyment of the satisfaction of craving is only a vital and physical degradation of the will to delight. It is essential that we should distinguish between pure will and desire, between the inner will to delight and the outer lust and craving of the mind and body. If we are unable to make this distinction practically in the experience of our being, we can only make a choice between a life-killing asceticism and the gross will to live or else try to effect an awkward, uncertain and precarious compromise between them. This is in fact what the mass of men do; a small minority trample down the life instinct and strain after an ascetic perfection; most obey the gross will to live with such modifications and restraints as society imposes or the normal social man has been trained to impose on his own mind and actions; others set up a balance between ethical austerity and temperate indulgence of the desiring mental and vital self and see in this balance the golden mean of a sane mind and healthy human living. But none of these ways gives the perfection which we are seeking, the divine government of the will in life. To tread down altogether the prana, the vital being, is to kill the force of life by which the large action of the embodied soul in the human being must be supported; to indulge the gross will to live is to remain satisfied with imperfection; to compromise between them is to stop half way and possess neither earth nor heaven. But if we can get at the pure will undeformed by desire,—which we shall find to be a much more free, tranquil, steady and effective force than the leaping, smoke-stifled, soon fatigued and baffled flame of desire,—and at the calm inner will of delight not afflicted or limited by any trouble of craving, we can then transform the prana from a tyrant, enemy, assailant of the mind into an obedient instrument. We may call these greater things, too, by the name of desire, if we choose, but then we must suppose that there is a divine desire other than the vital craving, a God-desire of which this other and lower phenomenon is an obscure shadow and into which it has to be transfigured. It is better to keep distinct names for things which are entirely different in their character and inner action.

To rid the prana of desire and incidentally to reverse the ordinary poise of our nature and turn the vital being from a troublesomely dominant power into the obedient instrument of a free and unattached mind, is then the first step in purification. As this deformation of the psychical prana is corrected, the purification of the rest of the intermediary parts of the *antaḥkaraṇa* is facilitated, and when that correction is completed, their purification too can be easily made absolute. These intermediary parts are the emotional mind, the receptive sensational mind and the active sensational mind or mind of dynamic impulse. They all hang together in a strongly knotted interaction. The deformation of the emotional mind hinges upon the duality of liking and disliking, *rāga-dveṣa*, emotional attraction and repulsion. All the complexity of our emotions and their tyranny over the soul arise from the habitual responses of the soul of desire in the emotions and sensations to these attractions and repulsions. Love and hatred, hope and fear, grief and joy all have their founts in this one source. We like, love, welcome, hope for, joy in whatever our nature, the first habit of our being, or else a formed (often perverse) habit, the second nature of our being, presents to the mind as pleasant, *priyam*; we hate, dislike, fear, have repulsion from or grief of whatever it presents to us as unpleasant, *apriyam*. This habit of the emotional nature gets into the way of the intelligent will and makes it often a helpless slave of the emotional being or at least prevents it from exercising a free judgment and government of the nature. This deformation has to be corrected. By getting rid of desire in the psychic prana and its intermiscence in the emotional mind, we facilitate the correction. For then attachment which is the strong bond of the heart, falls away from the heart-strings; the involuntary habit of *rāga-dveṣa* remains, but, not being made obstinate by attachment, it can be dealt with more easily by the will and the intelligence. The restless heart can be conquered and get rid of the habit of attraction and repulsion.

But then if this is done, it may be thought, as with regard to desire, that this will be the death of the emotional being. It will certainly be so, if the deformation is eliminated but not replaced by the right action of the emotional mind; the mind will then pass into a neutral condition of blank indifference or into a luminous state of peaceful impartiality with no stir or wave of emotion. The former state is in no way desirable; the latter may be the perfection of a quietistic discipline, but in the integral perfection which does not reject love or shun various movement of delight, it can be no more than a stage which has to be overpassed, a preliminary passivity admitted as a first basis for a right activity. Attraction and repulsion, liking and disliking are a necessary mechanism for the normal man, they form a first principle of natural instinctive selection among the thousand flattering and formidable, helpful and dangerous impacts of the world around him. The buddhi starts with this material to work on and tries to correct the natural and instinctive by a wiser reasoned and willed selection; for obviously the pleasant is not always the right thing, the object to be preferred and selected, nor the unpleasant the wrong thing, the object to be shunned and rejected; the pleasant and the good, *preyas* and *śreyas*, have to be distinguished, and right reason has to choose and not the caprice of emotion. But this it can do much better when the emotional suggestion is withdrawn and the heart rests in a luminous passivity. Then too the right activity of the heart can be brought to the surface; for we find then that behind this emotion-ridden soul of desire there was waiting all the while a soul of love and lucid joy and delight, a pure psyche, which was clouded over by the deformations of anger, fear, hatred, repulsion and could not embrace the world with an impartial love and joy. But the purified heart is rid of anger, rid of fear, rid of hatred, rid of every shrinking and repulsion: it has a universal love, it can receive with an untroubled sweetness and clarity the various delight which God gives it in the world. But it is not the lax slave of love and delight; it does not desire, does not attempt to impose itself as the master of the actions. The selective process necessary to action is left principally to the buddhi and, when the buddhi has been overpassed, to the spirit in the supramental will, knowledge and Ananda.

The receptive sensational mind is the nervous mental basis of the affections; it receives mentally the impacts of things and gives to them the responses of mental pleasure and pain which are the starting-point of the duality of emotional liking and disliking. All the heart's emotions have a corresponding nervous-mental accompaniment, and we often find that when the heart is freed of any will to the dualities, there still survives a root of disturbance of nervous mind, or a memory in physical mind which falls more and more away to a quite physical character, the more it is repelled by the will in the buddhi. It becomes finally a mere suggestion from outside to which the nervous chords of the mind still occasionally respond until a complete purity liberates them into the same luminous universality of delight which the pure heart already possesses. The active dynamic mind of impulse is the lower organ or channel of responsive action; its deformation is a subjection to the suggestions of the impure emotional and sensational mentality and the desire of the prana, to impulses to action dictated by grief, fear, hatred, desire, lust, craving, and the rest of the unquiet brood. Its right form of action is a pure dynamic force of strength, courage, temperamental power, not acting for itself or in obedience to the lower members, but as an impartial channel for the dictates of the pure intelligence and will or the supramental Purusha. When we have got rid of these deformations and cleared the mentality for these truer forms of action, the lower mentality is purified and ready for perfection. But that perfection depends on the possession of a purified and enlightened buddhi; for the buddhi is the chief power in the mental being and the chief mental instrument of the Purusha.

# PURIFICATION — INTELLIGENCE AND WILL

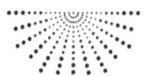

TO PURIFY the buddhi we must first understand its rather complex composition. And first we have to make clear the distinction, ignored in ordinary speech, between the *manas*, mind, and *buddhi*, the discerning intelligence and the enlightened will. Manas is the sense mind. Man's initial mentality is not at all a thing of reason and will; it is an animal, physical or sense mentality which constitutes its whole experience from the impressions made on it by the external world and by its own embodied consciousness which responds to the outward stimulus of this kind of experience. The buddhi only comes in as a secondary power which has in the evolution taken the first place, but is still dependent on the inferior instrument it uses; it depends for its workings on the sense mind and does what it can on its own higher range by a difficult, elaborate and rather stumbling extension of knowledge and action from the physical or sense basis. A half-enlightened physical or sense mentality is the ordinary type of the mind of man.

In fact the manas is a development from the external chitta; it is a first organising of the crude stuff of the consciousness excited and aroused by external contacts, *bāhya-sparśa*. What we are physically is a soul asleep in matter which has evolved to the partial wakefulness of a living body pervaded by a crude stuff of external consciousness more or less alive and attentive to the outward impacts of the external world in which we are developing our conscious being. In the animal this stuff of externalised consciousness organises itself into a well-regulated mental sense or organ of perceiving and acting mind. Sense is in fact the mental contact of the embodied consciousness with its surroundings. This contact is always essentially a mental phenomenon; but in fact it depends chiefly upon the development of certain physical organs of contact with objects and with their properties to whose images it is able by habit to give their mental values. What we call the physical senses have a double element, the physical-nervous impression of the object and the mental-nervous value we give to it, and the two together make up our seeing, hearing, smell, taste, touch with all those varieties of sensation of which they, and the touch chiefly, are the starting-point or first transmitting agency. But the manas is able to receive sense impressions and draw results from them by a direct transmission not dependent on the physical organ. This is more distinct in the lower creation. Man, though he has really a greater capacity for this direct sense, the sixth sense in the mind, has let it fall into abeyance by an exclusive reliance on the physical senses supplemented by the activity of the buddhi.

The manas is therefore in the first place an organiser of sense experience; in addition it organises the natural reactions of the will in the embodied consciousness and uses the body as an instrument, uses, as it is ordinarily put, the organs of action. This natural action too has a double element, a physico-nervous impulse and behind it a mental-nervous power-value of instinctive will-impulse. That makes up the nexus of first perceptions and actions which is common to all developing animal life. But in addition there is in the manas or sense-mind a first resulting thought-element which accompanies the operations of animal life. Just as the living body has a certain pervading and possessing action of consciousness, *citta*, which forms into this sense-mind, so the sense-mind has in it a certain pervading and possessing power which mentally uses the sense data, turns them into perceptions and first ideas, associates experience with other experiences, and in some way or other thinks and feels and wills on the sense basis.

This sensational thought-mind which is based upon sense, memory, association, first ideas and resultant generalisations or secondary ideas, is common to all developed animal life and mentality. Man indeed has given it an immense development and range and complexity impossible to the animal, but still, if he stopped there, he would only be a more highly effective animal. He gets beyond the animal range and height because he has been able to disengage and separate to a greater or less extent his thought action from the sense mentality, to draw back from the latter and observe its data and to act on it from above by a separated and partially freed intelligence. The intelligence and will of the animal are involved in the sense-mind and therefore altogether governed by it and carried on its stream of sensations, sense-perceptions, impulses; it is instinctive. Man is able to use a reason and will, a self-observing, thinking and all-observing, an intelligently willing mind which is no longer involved in the sense-mind, but acts from above and behind it in its own right, with a certain separateness and freedom. He is reflective, has a certain relative freedom of intelligent will. He has liberated in himself and has formed into a separate power the buddhi.

But what is this buddhi? From the point of view of Yogic knowledge we may say that it is that instrument of the soul, of the inner conscious being in nature, of the Purusha, by which it comes into some kind of conscious and ordered possession both of itself and its surroundings.

Behind all the action of the chitta and manas there is this soul, this Purusha; but in the lower forms of life it is mostly subconscient, asleep or half-awake, absorbed in the mechanical action of Nature; but it becomes more and more awake and comes more and more forward as it rises in the scale of life. By the activity of the buddhi it begins the process of an entire awakening. In the lower actions of the mind the soul suffers Nature rather than possesses her; for it is there entirely a slave to the mechanism which has brought it into conscious embodied experience. But in the buddhi we get to something, still a natural instrumentation, by which yet Nature seems to be helping and arming the Purusha to understand, possess and master her.

Neither understanding, possession nor mastery is complete, either because the buddhi in us is itself still incomplete, only yet half developed and half formed, or because it is in its nature only an intermediary instrument and before we can get complete knowledge and mastery, we must rise to something greater than the buddhi. Still it is a movement by which we come to the knowledge that there is a power within us greater than the animal life, a truth greater than the first truths or appearances perceived by the sense-mind, and can try to get at that truth and to labour towards a greater and more successful power of action and control, a more effective government both of our own nature and the nature of things around us, a higher knowledge, a higher power, a higher and larger enjoyment, a more exalted range of being. What then is the final object of this trend? Evidently, it must be for the Purusha to get to the highest and fullest truth of itself and of things, greatest truth of soul or self and greatest truth of Nature, and to an action and a status of being which shall be the result of or identical with that Truth, the power of this greatest knowledge and the enjoyment of that greatest being and consciousness to which it opens. This must be the final result of the evolution of the conscious being in Nature.

To arrive then at the whole truth of our self and Spirit and the knowledge, greatness, bliss of our free and complete being must be the object of the purification, liberation and perfection of the buddhi. But it is a common idea that this means not the full possession of Nature by the Purusha, but a rejection of Nature. We are to get at self by the removal of the action of Prakriti. As the buddhi, coming to the knowledge that the sense-mind only gives us appearances in which the soul is subject to Nature, discovers more real truths behind them, the soul must arrive at this knowledge that the buddhi too, when turned upon Nature, can give us only appearances and enlarge the subjection, and must discover behind them the pure truth of the Self. The Self is something quite other than Nature and the buddhi must purify itself of attachment to and preoccupation with natural things; so only can it discern and separate from them the pure Self and Spirit: the knowledge of the pure Self and Spirit is the only real knowledge, Ananda of the pure Self and Spirit is the only spiritual enjoyment, the consciousness and being of the pure Self and Spirit are the only real consciousness and being. Action and will must cease because all action is of the Nature; the will to be pure Self and Spirit means the cessation of all will to action.

But while the possession of the being, consciousness, delight, power of the Self is the condition of perfection,—for it is only by knowing and possessing and living in the truth of itself that the soul can become free and perfect,—we hold that Nature is an eternal action and manifestation of the Spirit; Nature is not a devil's trap, a set of misleading appearances created by desire, sense, life and mental will and intelligence, but these phenomena are hints and indications and behind all of them is a truth of Spirit which exceeds and uses them. We hold that there must be an inherent spiritual gnosis and will by which the secret Spirit in all knows its own truth, wills, manifests and governs its own being in Nature; to arrive at that, at communion with it or participation in it, must be part of our perfection. The object of the purification of the buddhi will then be to arrive at the possession of our own truth of self-being, but also at the possession of the highest truth of our being in Nature. For that purpose we must first purify the buddhi of all that makes it subject to the sense-mind and, that once done, purify it from its own limitations and convert its inferior mental intelligence and will into the greater action of a spiritual will and knowledge.

The movement of the buddhi to exceed the limits of the sense-mind is an effort already half accomplished in the human evolution; it is part of the common operation of Nature in man. The original action of the thought-mind, the intelligence and will in man, is a subject action. It accepts the evidence of the senses, the commands of the life-cravings, instincts, desires, emotions, the impulses of the dynamic sense-mind and only tries to give them a more orderly direction and effective success. But the man whose reason and will are led and dominated by the lower mind, is an inferior type of human nature, and the part of our conscious being which consents to this domination is the lowest part of our manhood. The higher action of the buddhi is to exceed and control the lower mind, not indeed to get rid of it, but to raise all the action of which it is the first suggestion into the nobler plane of will and intelligence. The impressions of the sense-mind are used by a thought which exceeds them and which arrives at truths they do not give, ideative truths of thought, truths of philosophy and science; a thinking, discovering, philosophic mind overcomes, rectifies and dominates the first mind of sense impressions. The impulsive reactive sensational mentality, the life-cravings and the mind of emotional desire are taken up by the intelligent will and are overcome, are rectified and dominated by a greater ethical mind which discovers and sets over them a law of right impulse, right desire, right emotion and right action. The receptive, crudely enjoying sensational mentality, the emotional mind and life mind are taken up by the intelligence and are overcome, rectified and dominated by a deeper, happier aesthetic mind which discovers and sets above them a law of true delight and beauty. All these new formations are used by a general Power of the intellectual, thinking and willing man in a soul of governing intellect, imagination, judgment, memory, volition, discerning reason and ideal feeling which uses them for knowledge, self-development, experience, discovery, creation, effectuation, aspires, strives, inwardly attains, endeavours to make a higher thing of the life of the soul in Nature. The primitive desire-soul no longer governs the being. It is still a desire-soul, but it is repressed and governed by a higher power, something which has manifested in itself the godheads of Truth, Will, Good, Beauty and tries to subject life to them. The crude desire-soul and mind is trying to convert itself into an ideal soul and mind, and the proportion in which some effect and harmony of this greater conscious being has been found and enthroned, is the measure of our increasing humanity.

But this is still a very incomplete movement. We find that it progresses towards a greater completeness in proportion as we arrive at two kinds of perfection; first, a greater and greater detachment from the control of the lower suggestions; secondly, an increasing discovery of a self-existent Being, Light, Power and Ananda which surpasses and transforms the normal humanity. The ethical mind becomes perfect in proportion as it detaches itself from desire, sense suggestion, impulse, customary dictated action and discovers a self of Right, Love, Strength and Purity in which it can live accomplished and make it the foundation of all its actions. The aesthetic mind is perfected in proportion as it detaches itself from all its cruder pleasures and from outward conventional canons of the aesthetic reason and discovers a self-existent self and spirit of pure and infinite Beauty and Delight which gives its own light and joy to the material of the aesthesis. The mind of knowledge is perfected when it gets away from impression and dogma and opinion and discovers a light of self-knowledge and intuition which illumines all the workings of the sense and reason, all self-experience and world-experience. The will is perfected when it gets away from and behind its impulses and its customary ruts of effectuation and discovers an inner power of the Spirit which is the source of an intuitive and luminous action and an original harmonious creation. The movement of perfection is away from all domination by the lower nature and towards a pure and powerful reflection of the being, power, knowledge and delight of the Spirit and Self in the buddhi.

The Yoga of self-perfection is to make this double movement as absolute as possible. All immiscence of desire in the buddhi is an impurity. The intelligence coloured by desire is an impure intelligence and it distorts Truth; the will coloured by desire is an impure will and it puts a stamp of distortion, pain and imperfection upon the soul's activity. All immiscence of the emotions of the soul of desire is an impurity and similarly distorts both the knowledge and the action. All subjection of the buddhi to the sensations and impulses is an impurity. The thought and will have to stand back detached from desire, troubling emotion, distracting or mastering impulse and to act in their own right until they can discover a greater guide, a Will, Tapas or divine Shakti which will take the place of desire and mental will and impulse, an Ananda or pure delight of the spirit and an illumined spiritual knowledge which will express themselves in the action of that Shakti. This complete detachment, impossible without an entire self-government, equality, calm, *śama, samatā, śānti*, is the surest step towards the purification of the buddhi. A calm, equal and detached mind can alone reflect the peace or base the action of the liberated spirit.

The buddhi itself is burdened with a mixed and impure action. When we reduce it to its own proper forms, we find that it has three stages or elevations of its functioning. First, its lowest basis is a habitual, customary action which is a link between the higher reason and the sense-mind, a kind of current understanding. This understanding is in itself dependent on the witness of the senses and the rule of action which the reason deduces from the sense-mind's perception of and attitude to life. It is not capable of itself forming pure thought and will, but it takes the workings of the higher reason and turns them into coin of opinion and customary standard of thought or canon of action. When we perform a sort of practical analysis of the thinking mind, cut away this element and hold back the higher reason free, observing and silent, we find that this current understanding begins to run about in a futile circle, repeating all its formed opinions and responses to the impressions of things, but incapable of any strong adaptation and initiation. As it feels more and more the refusal of sanction from the higher reason, it begins to fail, to lose confidence in itself and its forms and habits, to distrust the intellectual action and to fall into weakness and silence. The stilling of this current, running, circling, repeating thought-mind is the principal part of that silencing of the thought which is one of the most effective disciplines of Yoga.

But the higher reason itself has a first stage of dynamic, pragmatic intellectuality in which creation, action and will are the real motive and thought and knowledge are employed to form basic constructions and suggestions which are used principally for effectuation. To this pragmatic reason truth is only a formation of the intellect effective for the action of the inner and the outer life. When we cut it away from the still higher reason which seeks impersonally to reflect Truth rather than to create personally effective truth, we find then that this pragmatic reason can originate, progress, enlarge the experience by dynamic knowledge, but it has to depend on the current understanding as a pedestal and base and put its whole weight on life and becoming. It is in itself therefore a mind of the Will to life and action, much more a mind of Will than a mind of knowledge: it does not live in any assured and constant and eternal Truth, but in progressing and changing aspects of Truth which serve the shifting forms of our life and becoming or, at the highest, help life to grow and progress. By itself this pragmatic mind can give us no firm foundation and no fixed goal; it lives in the truth of the hour, not in any truth of eternity. But when purified of dependence on the customary understanding, it is a great creator and in association with the highest mental reason it becomes a strong channel and bold servant for the effectuation of Truth in life. The value of its work will depend on the value and the power of the highest truth-seeking reason. But by itself it is a sport of Time and a bond-slave of Life. The seeker of the Silence has to cast it away from him; the seeker of the integral Divinity has to pass beyond it, to replace and transform this thinking mind intent on Life by a greater effectuating spiritual Will, the Truth-Will of the spirit.

The third and noblest stage of the intellectual will and reason is an intelligence which seeks for some universal reality or for a still higher self-existent Truth for its own sake and tries to live in that Truth. This is primarily a mind of knowledge and only secondarily a mind of Will. In its excess of tendency it often becomes incapable of Will except the one will to know; for action it is dependent on the aid of the pragmatic mind and therefore man tends in action to fall away from the purity of the Truth his highest knowledge holds into a mixed, inferior, inconstant and impure effectuation. The disparity, even when it is not an opposition, between knowledge and will is one of the principal defects of the human buddhi. But there are other inherent limitations of all human thinking. This highest Buddhi does not work in man in its own purity; it is assailed by the defects of the lower mentality, continually clouded by it, distorted, veiled, and prevented or lamed in its own proper action. Purified as much as may be from that habit of mental degradation, the human buddhi is still a power that searches for the Truth, but is never in full or direct possession of it; it can only reflect truth of the spirit and try to make it its own by giving it a limited mental value and a distinct mental body. Nor does it reflect integrally, but seizes either an uncertain totality or else a sum of limited particulars. First it seizes on this or that partial reflection and by subjection to the habit of customary mind turns it into a fixed imprisoning opinion; all new truth it judges from the standpoint it has thus formed and therefore puts on it the colour of a limiting prejudgment. Release it as much as possible from this habit of limiting opinion, still it is subject to another affliction, the demand of the pragmatic mind for immediate effectuation, which gives it no time to proceed to larger truth, but fixes it by the power of effective realisation in whatever it has already judged, known and lived. Freed from all these chains, the buddhi can become a pure and flexible reflector of Truth, adding light to light, proceeding from realisation to realisation. It is then limited only by its own inherent limitations.

These limitations are mainly of two kinds. First, its realisations are only mental realisations; to get to the Truth itself we have to go beyond the mental buddhi. Again, the nature of the mind prevents it from making an effective unification of the truths it seizes. It can only put them side by side and see oppositions or effect some kind of partial, executive and practical combination. But it finds finally that the aspects of the Truth are infinite and that none of its intellectual forms are quite valid, because the spirit is infinite and in the spirit all is true, but nothing in the mind can give the whole truth of the spirit. Either then the buddhi becomes a pure mirror of many reflections, reflecting all truth that falls on it, but ineffective and when turned to action either incapable of decision or chaotic, or it has to make a selection and act as if that partiality were the whole truth, though it knows otherwise. It acts in a helpless limitation of Ignorance, though it may hold a Truth far greater than its action. On the other hand, it may turn away from life and thought and seek to exceed itself and pass into the Truth beyond it. This it may do by seizing on some aspect, some principle, some symbol or suggestion of reality and pushing that to its absolute, all-absorbing, all-excluding term of realisation or by seizing on and realising some idea of indeterminate Being or Non-Being from which all thought and life fall away into cessation. The buddhi casts itself into a luminous sleep and the soul passes away into some ineffable height of spiritual being.

Therefore in dealing with the buddhi, we must either take one of these choices or else try the rarer adventure of lifting the soul from the mental being into the spiritual gnosis to see what we can find in the very core of that supernal light and power. This gnosis contains the sun of the divine Knowledge-Will burning in the heavens of the supreme conscious Being, to which the mental intelligence and will are only a focus of diffused and deflected rays and reflections. That possesses the divine unity and yet or rather therefore can govern the multiplicity and diversity: whatever selection, self-limitation, combination it makes is not imposed on it by Ignorance, but is self-developed by a power of self-possessing divine Knowledge. When the gnosis is gained, it can then be turned on the whole nature to divinise the human being. It is impossible to rise into it at once; if that could be done, it would mean a sudden and violent overshooting, a breaking or slipping through the gates of the Sun, *sūryasya dvārā*, without near possibility of return. We have to form as a link or bridge an intuitive or illuminated mind, which is not the direct gnosis, but in which a first derivative body of the gnosis can form. This illumined mind will first be a mixed power which we shall have to purify of all its mental dependence and mental forms so as to convert all willing and thinking into thought-sight and truth-seeing will by an illumined discrimination, intuition, inspiration, revelation. That will be the final purification of the intelligence and the preparation for the siddhi of the gnosis.

# THE LIBERATION OF THE SPIRIT

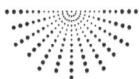

THE PURIFICATION of the mental being and the psychic prana —we will leave aside for the time the question of the physical purification, that of the body and physical prana, though that too is necessary to an integral perfection,—prepares the ground for a spiritual liberation. *śuddhi* is the condition for *mukti*. All purification is a release, a delivery; for it is a throwing away of limiting, binding, obscuring imperfections and confusions: purification from desire brings the freedom of the psychic prana, purification from wrong emotions and troubling reactions the freedom of the heart, purification from the obscuring limited thought of the sense mind the freedom of the intelligence, purification from mere intellectuality the freedom of the gnosis. But all this is an instrumental liberation. The freedom of the soul, *mukti*, is of a larger and more essential character; it is an opening out of mortal limitation into the illimitable immortality of the Spirit.

For certain ways of thinking liberation is a throwing off of all nature, a silent state of pure being, a nirvana or extinction, a dissolution of the natural existence into some indefinable Absolute, *mokṣa*. But an absorbed and immersed bliss, a wideness of action-less peace, a release of self-extinction or a self-drowning in the Absolute is not our aim. We shall give to the idea of liberation, *mukti*, only the connotation of that inner change which is common to all experience of this kind, essential to perfection and indispensable to spiritual freedom. We shall find that it then implies always two things, a rejection and an assumption, a negative and a positive side; the negative movement of freedom is a liberation from the principal bonds, the master-knots of the lower soul-nature, the positive side an opening or growth into the higher spiritual existence. But what are these master-knots—other and deeper twistings than the instrumental knots of the mind, heart, psychic life-force? We find them pointed out for us and insisted on with great force and a constant emphatic repetition in the Gita; they are four, desire, ego, the dualities and the three gunas of Nature; for to be desireless, ego-less, equal of mind and soul and spirit and *nistraiguṇya*, is in the idea of the Gita to be free, *mukta*. We may accept this description; for everything essential is covered by its amplitude. On the other hand, the positive sense of freedom is to be universal in soul, transcendently one in spirit with God, possessed of the highest divine nature,—as we may say, like to God, or one with him in the law of our being. This is the whole and full sense of liberation and this is the integral freedom of the spirit.

We have already had to speak of purification from the psychic desire of which the craving of the prana is the evolutionary or, as we may put it, the practical basis. But this is in the mental and psychic nature; spiritual desirelessness has a wider and more essential meaning: for desire has a double knot, a lower knot in the prana, which is a craving in the instruments, and a very subtle knot in the soul itself with the buddhi as its first support or *pratiṣṭhā*, which is the inmost origin of this mesh of our bondage. When we look from below, desire presents itself to us as a craving of the life force which subtilises in the emotions into a craving of the heart and is farther subtilised in the intelligence into a craving, preference, passion of the aesthetic, ethical, dynamic or rational turn of the buddhi. This desire is essential to the ordinary man; he cannot live or act as an individual without knotting up all his action into the service of some kind of lower or higher craving, preference or passion. But when we are able to look at desire from above, we see that what supports this instrumental desire is a will of the spirit. There is a will, *tapas*, *śakti*, by which the secret spirit imposes on its outer members all their action and draws from it an active delight of its being, an ananda, in which they very obscurely and imperfectly, if at all consciously, partake. This tapas is the will of the transcendent spirit who creates the universal movement, of the universal spirit who supports and informs it, of the free individual spirit who is the soul centre of its multiplicities. It is one will, free in all these at once, comprehensive, harmonious, unified; we find it, when we live and act in the spirit, to be an effortless and desireless, a spontaneous and illumined, a self-fulfilling and self-possessing, a satisfied and blissful will of the spiritual delight of being.

But the moment the individual soul leans away from the universal and transcendent truth of its being, leans towards ego, tries to make this will a thing of its own, a separate personal energy, that will changes its character: it becomes an effort, a straining, a heat of force which may have its fiery joys of effectuation and of possession, but has also its afflicting recoils and pain of labour. It is this that turns in each instrument into an intellectual, emotional, dynamic, sensational or vital will of desire, wish, craving. Even when the instruments *per se* are purified of their own apparent initiative and particular kind of desire, this imperfect tapas may still remain, and so long as it conceals the source or deforms the type of the inner action, the soul has not the bliss of liberty, or can only have it by refraining from all action; even, if allowed to persist, it will rekindle the pranic or other desires or at least throw a reminiscent shadow of them on the being. This spiritual seed or beginning of desire too must be expelled, renounced, cast away: the sadhaka must either choose an active peace and complete inner silence or lose individual initiation, *saṅkalpārambha*, in a unity with the universal will, the tapas of the divine Shakti. The passive way is to be inwardly immobile, without effort, wish, expectation or any turn to action, *niśceṣṭa, anīha, nirapekṣa, nivṛtta*; the active way is to be thus immobile and impersonal in the mind, but to allow the supreme Will in its spiritual purity to act through the purified instruments. Then, if the soul abides on the level of the spiritualised mentality, it becomes an instrument only, but is itself without initiative or action, *niṣkriya, sarvārambha-parityāgī*. But if it rises to the gnosis, it is at once an instrument and a participant in the bliss of the divine action and the bliss of the divine Ananda; it unifies in itself the *prakṛti* and the *puruṣa*.

The ego turn, the separative turn of the being, is the fulcrum of the whole embarrassed labour of the ignorance and the bondage. So long as one is not free from the ego sense, there can be no real freedom. The seat of the ego is said to be in the buddhi; it is an ignorance of the discriminating mind and reason which discriminate wrongly and take the individuation of mind, life and body for a truth of separative existence and are turned away from the greater reconciling truth of the oneness of all existence. At any rate in man it is the ego idea which chiefly supports the falsehood of a separative existence; to get rid of this idea, to dwell on the opposite idea of unity, of the one self, the one spirit, the one being of nature is therefore an effective remedy; but it is not by itself absolutely effective. For the ego, though it supports itself by this ego idea, *ahambuddhi*, finds its most powerful means for a certain obstinacy or passion of persistence in the normal action of the sense-mind, the prana and the body. To cast out of us the ego idea is not entirely possible or not entirely effective until these instruments have undergone purification; for, their action being persistently egoistic and separative, the buddhi is carried away by them,—as a boat by winds on the sea, says the Gita,—the knowledge in the intelligence is being constantly obscured or lost temporarily and has to be restored again, a very labour of Sisyphus. But if the lower instruments have been purified of egoistic desire, wish, will, egoistic passion, egoistic emotion and the buddhi itself of egoistic idea and preference, then the knowledge of the spiritual truth of oneness can find a firm foundation. Till then, the ego takes all sorts of subtle forms and we imagine ourselves to be free from it, when we are really acting as its instruments and all we have attained is a certain intellectual poise which is not the true spiritual liberation. Moreover, to throw away the active sense of ego is not enough; that may merely bring an inactive state of the mentality, a certain passive inert quietude of separate being may take the place of the kinetic egoism, which is also not the true liberation. The ego sense must be replaced by a oneness with the transcendental Divine and with universal being.

This necessity arises from the fact that the buddhi is only a *pratiṣṭhā* or chief support of the ego-sense in its manifold play, *ahaṅkāra*; but in its source it is a degradation or deformation of a truth of our spiritual being. The truth of being is that there is a transcendent existence, supreme self or spirit, a timeless soul of existence, an eternal, a Divine, or even we may speak of it in relation to current mental ideas of the Godhead as a supra-Divine, which is here immanent, all-embracing, all-initiating and all-governing, a great universal Spirit; and the individual is a conscious power of being of the Eternal, capable eternally of relations with him, but one with him too in the very core of reality of its own eternal existence. This is a truth which the intelligence can apprehend, can, when once purified, reflect, transmit, hold in a derivative fashion, but it can only be entirely realised, lived and made effective in the spirit. When we live in the spirit, then we not only know, but are this truth of our being. The individual then enjoys in the spirit, in the bliss of the spirit, his oneness with the universal existence, his oneness with the timeless Divine and his oneness with all other beings and that is the essential sense of a spiritual liberation from the ego. But the moment the soul leans towards the mental limitation, there is a certain sense of spiritual separativeness which has its joys, but may at any moment lapse into the entire ego-sense, ignorance, oblivion of oneness. To get rid of this separativeness an attempt is made to absorb oneself in the idea and realisation of the Divine, and this takes in certain forms of spiritual askesis the turn of a strain towards the abolition of all individual being and a casting away, in the trance of immersion, of all individual or universal relations with the Divine, in others it becomes an absorbed dwelling in him and not in this world or a continual absorbed or intent living in his presence, *sāyujya, sālokya, sāmīpya mukti*. The way proposed for the integral Yoga is a lifting up and surrender of the whole being to him, by which not only do we become one with him in our spiritual existence, but dwell too in him and he in us, so that the whole nature is full of his presence and changed into the divine nature; we become one spirit and consciousness and life and substance with the Divine and at the same time we live and move in and have a various joy of that oneness. This integral liberation from the ego into the divine spirit and nature can only be relatively complete on our present level, but it begins to become absolute as we open to and mount into the gnosis. This is the liberated perfection. The liberation from ego, the liberation from desire together found the central spiritual freedom. The sense, the idea, the experience that I am a separately self-existent being in the universe, and the forming of consciousness and force of being into the mould of that experience are the root of all suffering, ignorance and evil. And it is so because that falsifies both in practice and in cognition the whole real truth of things; it limits the being, limits the consciousness, limits the power of our being, limits the bliss of being; this limitation again produces a wrong way of existence, wrong way of consciousness, wrong way of using the power of our being and consciousness, and wrong, perverse and contrary forms of the delight of existence. The soul limited in being and self-isolated in its environment feels itself no longer in unity and harmony with its Self, with God, with the universe, with all around it; but rather it finds itself at odds with the universe, in conflict and disaccord with other beings who are its other selves, but whom it treats as not-self; and so long as this disaccord and disagreement last, it cannot possess its world and it cannot enjoy the universal life, but is full of unease, fear, afflictions of all kinds, in a painful struggle to preserve and increase itself and possess its surroundings,—for to possess its world is the nature of infinite spirit and the necessary urge in all being. The satisfactions it gets from this labour and effort are of a stinted, perverse and unsatisfying kind: for the one real satisfaction it has is that of growth, of an increasing return towards itself, of some realisation of accord and harmony, of successful self-creation and self-realisation, but the little of these things that it can achieve on the basis of ego-consciousness is always limited, insecure, imperfect, transitory. It is at war too with its own self,—first because, since it is no longer in possession of the central harmonising truth of its own being, it cannot properly control its natural members or accord their tendencies, powers and demands; it has not the secret of harmony, because it has not the secret of its own unity and self-possession; and, secondly, not being in possession of its highest self, it has to struggle towards that, is not allowed to be at peace till it is in possession of its own true highest being. All this means that it is not at one with God; for to be at one with God is to be at one with oneself, at one with the universe and at one with all beings. This oneness is the secret of a right and a divine existence. But the ego cannot have it, because it is in its very nature separative and because even with regard to ourselves, to our own psychological existence it is a false centre of unity; for it tries to find the unity of our being in an identification with a shifting mental, vital, physical personality, not with the eternal self of our total existence. Only in the spiritual self can we possess the true unity; for there the individual enlarges to his own total being and finds himself one with universal existence and with the transcending Divinity.

All the trouble and suffering of the soul proceeds from this wrong egoistic and separative way of existence. The soul not in possession of its free self-existence, *anātmavān*, because it is limited in its consciousness, is limited in knowledge; and this limited knowledge takes the form of a falsifying knowledge. The struggle to return to a true knowing is imposed upon it, but the ego in the separative mind is satisfied with shows and fragments of knowledge which it pieces together into some false or some imperfect total or governing notion, and this knowledge fails it and has to be abandoned for a fresh pursuit of the one thing to be known. That one thing is the Divine, the Self, the Spirit in whom universal and individual being find at last their right foundation and their right harmonies. Again, because it is limited in force, the ego-prisoned soul is full of many incapacities; wrong knowledge is accompanied by wrong will, wrong tendencies and impulses of the being, and the acute sense of this wrongness is the root of the human consciousness of sin. This deficiency of its nature it tries to set right by standards of conduct which will help it to remove the egoistic consciousness and satisfactions of sin by the egoistic consciousness and self-satisfaction of virtue, the rajasic by the sattwic egoism. But the original sin has to be cured, the separation of its being and will from the divine Being and the divine Will; when it returns to unity with the divine Will and Being, it rises beyond sin and virtue to the infinite self-existent purity and the security of its own divine nature.

Its incapacities it tries to set right by organising its imperfect knowledge and disciplining its half-enlightened will and force and directing them by some systematic effort of the reason; but the result must always be a limited, uncertain, mutable and stumbling way and standard of capacity in action. Only when it returns again to the large unity of the free spirit, *bhūmā*, can the action of its nature move perfectly as the instrument of the infinite Spirit and in the steps of the Right and Truth and Power which belong to the free soul acting from the supreme centre of its existence. Again, because it is limited in the delight of being, it is unable to lay hold on the secure, self-existent perfect bliss of the spirit or the delight, the Ananda of the universe which keeps the world in motion, but is only able to move in a mixed and shifting succession of pleasures and pains, joys and sorrows, or must take refuge in some conscient inconscience or neutral indifference. The ego mind cannot do otherwise, and the soul which has externalised itself in ego, is subjected to this unsatisfactory, secondary, imperfect, often perverse, troubled or annulled enjoyment of existence; yet all the time the spiritual and universal Ananda is within, in the self, in the spirit, in its secret unity with God and existence. To cast away the chain of ego and go back to free self, immortal spiritual being is the soul's return to its own eternal divinity.

The will to the imperfect separative being, that wrong Tapas which makes the soul in Nature attempt to individualise itself, to individualise its being, consciousness, force of being, delight of existence in a separative sense, to have these things as its own, in its own right, and not in the right of God and of the universal oneness, is that which brings about this wrong turn and creates the ego. To turn from this original desire is therefore essential, to get back to the will without desire whose whole enjoyment of being and whole will in being is that of a free universal and unifying Ananda. These two things are one, liberation from the will that is of the nature of desire and liberation from the ego, and the oneness which is brought about by the happy loss of the will of desire and the ego, is the essence of Mukti.

# THE LIBERATION OF THE NATURE

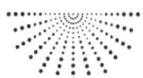

THE TWO sides of our being, conscious experiencing soul and executive Nature continuously and variously offering to the soul her experiences, determine in their meeting all the affections of our inner status and its responses. Nature contributes the character of the happenings and the forms of the instruments of experience, the soul meets it by an assent to the natural determinations of the response to these happenings or by a will to other determination which it imposes upon the nature. The acceptance of the instrumental ego consciousness and the will to desire are the initial consent of the self to the lapse into the lower ranges of experience in which it forgets its divine nature of being; the rejection of these things, the return to free self and the will of the divine delight in being is the liberation of the spirit. But on the other side stand the contributions of Nature herself to the mixed tangle, which she imposes on the soul's experience of her doings and makings when once that first initial consent has been given and made the law of the whole outward transaction. Nature's essential contributions are two, the gunas and the dualities. This inferior action of Nature in which we live has certain essential qualitative modes which constitute the whole basis of its inferiority. The constant effect of these modes on the soul in its natural powers of mind, life and body is a discordant and divided experience, a strife of opposites, *dvandva*, a motion in all its experience and an oscillation between or a mixture of constant pairs of contraries, of combining positives and negatives, dualities. A complete liberation from the ego and the will of desire must bring with it a superiority to the qualitative modes of the inferior Nature, *traiguṇyātītya*, a release from this mixed and discordant experience, a cessation or solution of the dual action of Nature. But on this side too there are two kinds of freedom. A liberation from Nature in a quiescent bliss of the spirit is the first form of release. A farther liberation of the Nature into a divine quality and spiritual power of world-experience fills the supreme calm with the supreme kinetic bliss of knowledge, power, joy and mastery. A divine unity of supreme spirit and its supreme nature is the integral liberation.

Nature, because she is a power of spirit, is essentially qualitative in her action. One may almost say that Nature is only the power in being and the development in action of the infinite qualities of the spirit, *anantaguṇa*. All else belongs to her outward and more mechanical aspects; but this play of quality is the essential thing, of which the rest is the result and mechanical combination. Once we have set right the working of the essential power and quality, all the rest becomes subject to the control of the experiencing Purusha. But in the inferior nature of things the play of infinite quality is subject to a limited measure, a divided and conflicting working, a system of opposites and discords between which some practical mobile system of concords has to be found and to be kept in action; this play of concorded discords, conflicting qualities, disparate powers and ways of experience compelled to some just manageable, partial, mostly precarious agreement, an unstable mutable equilibrium, is managed by a fundamental working in three qualitative modes which conflict and combine together in all her creations. These three modes have been given in the Sankhya system, which is generally adopted for this purpose by all the schools of philosophic thought and of Yoga in India, the three names, *sattva, rajas* and *tamas*.[1] Tamas is the principle and power of inertia; rajas is the principle of kinesis, passion, endeavour, struggle, initiation (*ārambha*); sattwa the principle of assimilation, equilibrium and harmony. The metaphysical bearing of this classification does not concern us; but in its psychological and spiritual bearing it is of immense practical importance, because these three principles enter into all things, combine to give them their turn of active nature, result, effectuation, and their unequal working in the soul-experience is the constituent force of our active personality, our temperament, type of nature and cast of psychological response to experience. All character of action and experience in us is determined by the predominance and by the proportional interaction of these three qualities or modes of Nature. The soul in its personality is obliged, as it were, to run into their moulds; mostly, too, it is controlled by them rather than has any free control of them. The soul can only be free by rising above and rejecting the tormented strife of their unequal action and their insufficient concords and combinations and precarious harmonies, whether in the sense of a complete quiescence from the half-regulated chaos of their action or in the sense of a superiority to this lower turn of nature and a higher control or transformation of their working. There must be either an emptiness of the gunas or a superiority to the gunas.

The gunas affect every part of our natural being. They have indeed their strongest relative hold in the three different members of it, mind, life and body. Tamas, the principle of inertia, is strongest in material nature and in our physical being. The action of this principle is of two kinds, inertia of force and inertia of knowledge. Whatever is predominantly governed by Tamas, tends in its force to a sluggish inaction and immobility or else to a mechanical action which it does not possess, but is possessed by obscure forces which drive it in a mechanical round of energy; equally in its consciousness it turns to an inconscience or enveloped subconscience or to a reluctant, sluggish or in some way mechanical conscious action which does not possess the idea of its own energy, but is guided by an idea which seems external to it or at least concealed from its active awareness. Thus the principle of our body is in its nature inert, subconscient, incapable of anything but a mechanical and habitual self-guidance and action: though it has like everything else a principle of kinesis and a principle of equilibrium of its state and action, an inherent principle of response and a secret consciousness, the greatest portion of its rajasic motions are contributed by the life-power and all the overt consciousness by the mental being. The principle of rajas has its strongest hold on the vital nature. It is the Life within us that is the strongest kinetic motor power, but the life-power in earthly beings is possessed by the force of desire, therefore rajas turns always to action and desire; desire is the strongest human and animal initiator of most kinesis and action, predominant to such an extent that many consider it the father of all action and even the originator of our being. Moreover, rajas finding itself in a world of matter which starts from the principle of inconscience and a mechanical driven inertia, has to work against an immense contrary force; therefore its whole action takes on the nature of an effort, a struggle, a besieged and an impeded conflict for possession which is distressed in its every step by a limiting incapacity, disappointment and suffering: even its gains are precarious and limited and marred by the reaction of the effort and an aftertaste of insufficiency and transience. The principle of sattwa has its strongest hold in the mind; not so much in the lower parts of the mind which are dominated by the rajasic life-power, but mostly in the intelligence and the will of the reason. Intelligence, reason, rational will are moved by the nature of their predominant principle towards a constant effort of assimilation, assimilation by knowledge, assimilation by a power of understanding will, a constant effort towards equilibrium, some stability, rule, harmony of the conflicting elements of natural happening and experience. This satisfaction it gets in various ways and in various degrees of acquisition. The attainment of assimilation, equilibrium and harmony brings with it always a relative but more or less intense and satisfying sense of ease, happiness, mastery, security, which is other than the troubled and vehement pleasures insecurely bestowed by the satisfaction of rajasic desire and passion. Light and happiness are the characteristics of the sattwic guna. The whole nature of the embodied living mental being is determined by these three gunas.

But these are only predominant powers in each part of our complex system. The three qualities mingle, combine and strive in every fibre and in every member of our intricate psychology. The mental character is made by them, the character of our reason, the character of our will, the character of our moral, aesthetic, emotional, dynamic, sensational being. Tamas brings in all the ignorance, inertia, weakness, incapacity which afflicts our nature, a clouded reason, nescience, unintelligence, a clinging to habitual notions and mechanical ideas, the refusal to think and know, the small mind, the closed avenues, the trotting round of mental habit, the dark and the twilit places. Tamas brings in the impotent will, want of faith and self-confidence and initiative, the disinclination to act, the shrinking from endeavour and aspiration, the poor and little spirit, and in our moral and dynamic being the inertia, the cowardice, baseness, sloth, lax subjection to small and ignoble motives, the weak yielding to our lower nature. Tamas brings into our emotional nature insensibility, indifference, want of sympathy and openness, the shut soul, the callous heart, the soon spent affection and languor of the feelings, into our aesthetic and sensational nature the dull aesthesis, the limited range of response, the insensibility to beauty, all that makes in man the coarse, heavy and vulgar spirit. Rajas contributes our normal active nature with all its good and evil; when unchastened by a sufficient element of sattwa, it turns to egoism, self-will and violence, the perverse, obstinate or exaggerating action of the reason, prejudice, attachment to opinion, clinging to error, the subservience of the intelligence to our desires and preferences and not to the truth, the fanatic or the sectarian mind, self-will, pride, arrogance, selfishness, ambition, lust, greed, cruelty, hatred, jealousy, the egoisms of love, all the vices and passions, the exaggerations of the aesthesis, the morbidities and perversions of the sensational and vital being. Tamas in its own right produces the coarse, dull and ignorant type of human nature, rajas the vivid, restless, kinetic man, driven by the breath of action, passion and desire. Sattwa produces a higher type. The gifts of sattwa are the mind of reason and balance, clarity of the disinterested truth-seeking open intelligence, a will subordinated to the reason or guided by the ethical spirit, self-control, equality, calm, love, sympathy, refinement, measure, fineness of the aesthetic and emotional mind, in the sensational being delicacy, just acceptivity, moderation and poise, a vitality subdued and governed by the mastering intelligence. The accomplished types of the sattwic man are the philosopher, saint and sage, of the rajasic man the statesman, warrior, forceful man of action. But in all men there is in greater or less proportions a mingling of the gunas, a multiple personality and in most a good deal of shifting and alternation from the predominance of one to the prevalence of another guna; even in the governing form of their nature most human beings are of a mixed type. All the colour and variety of life is made of the intricate pattern of the weaving of the gunas.

But richness of life, even a sattwic harmony of mind and nature does not constitute spiritual perfection. There is a relative possible perfection, but it is a perfection of incompleteness, some partial height, force, beauty, some measure of nobility and greatness, some imposed and precariously sustained balance. There is a relative mastery, but it is a mastery of the body by life or of the life by mind, not a free possession of the instruments by the liberated and self-possessing spirit. The gunas have to be transcended if we would arrive at spiritual perfection. Tamas evidently has to be overcome, inertia and ignorance and incapacity cannot be elements of a true perfection; but it can only be overcome in Nature by the force of rajas aided by an increasing force of sattwa. Rajas has to be overcome, egoism, personal desire and self-seeking passion are not elements of the true perfection; but it can only be overcome by force of sattwa enlightening the being and force of tamas limiting the action. Sattwa itself does not give the highest or the integral perfection; sattwa is always a quality of the limited nature; sattwic knowledge is the light of a limited mentality; sattwic will is the government of a limited intelligent force. Moreover, sattwa cannot act by itself in Nature, but has to rely for all action on the aid of rajas, so that even sattwic action is always liable to the imperfections of rajas; egoism, perplexity, inconsistency, a one-sided turn, a limited and exaggerated will, exaggerating itself in the intensity of its limitations, pursue the mind and action even of the saint, philosopher and sage. There is a sattwic as well as a rajasic or tamasic egoism, at the highest an egoism of knowledge or virtue; but the mind's egoism of whatever type is incompatible with liberation. All the three gunas have to be transcended. Sattwa may bring us near to the Light, but its limited clarity falls away from us when we enter into the luminous body of the divine Nature.

This transcendence is usually sought by a withdrawal from the action of the lower nature. That withdrawal brings with it a stressing of the tendency to inaction. Sattwa when it wishes to intensify itself, seeks to get rid of rajas and calls in the aid of the tamasic principle of inaction; that is the reason why a certain type of highly sattwic men live intensely in the inward being, but hardly at all in the outward life of action, or else are there incompetent and ineffective. The seeker of liberation goes farther in this direction, strives by imposing an enlightened tamas on his natural being, a tamas which by this saving enlightenment is more of a quiescence than an incapacity, to give the sattwic guna freedom to lose itself in the light of the spirit. A quietude and stillness is imposed on the body, on the active life-soul of desire and ego, on the external mind, while the sattwic nature by stress of meditation, by an exclusive concentration of adoration, by a will turned inward to the Supreme, strives to merge itself in the spirit. But if this is sufficient for a quietistic release, it is not sufficient for the freedom of an integral perfection. This liberation depends upon inaction and is not entirely self-existent and absolute; the moment the soul turns to action, it finds that the activity of the nature is still the old imperfect motion. There is a liberation of the soul from the nature which is gained by inaction, but not a liberation of the soul in nature perfect and self-existent whether in action or in inaction. The question then arises whether such a liberation and perfection are possible and what may be the condition of this perfect freedom.

The ordinary idea is that it is not possible because all action is of the lower gunas, necessarily defective, *sadoṣam*, caused by the motion, inequality, want of balance, unstable strife of the gunas; but when these unequal gunas fall into perfect equilibrium, all action of Nature ceases and the soul rests in its quietude. The divine Being, we may say, may either exist in his silence or act in Nature through her instrumentation, but in that case must put on the appearance of her strife and imperfection. That may be true of the ordinary deputed action of the Divine in the human spirit with its present relations of soul to nature in an embodied imperfect mental being, but it is not true of the divine nature of perfection. The strife of the gunas is only a representation in the imperfection of the lower nature; what the three gunas stand for are three essential powers of the Divine which are not merely existent in a perfect equilibrium of quietude, but unified in a perfect consensus of divine action. Tamas in the spiritual being becomes a divine calm, which is not an inertia and incapacity of action, but a perfect power, *śakti*, holding in itself all its capacity and capable of controlling and subjecting to the law of calm even the most stupendous and enormous activity: rajas becomes a self-effecting initiating sheer Will of the spirit, which is not desire, endeavour, striving passion, but the same perfect power of being, *śakti*, capable of an infinite, imperturbable and blissful action. Sattwa becomes not the modified mental light, *prakāśa*, but the self-existent light of the divine being, *jyotiḥ*, which is the soul of the perfect power of being and illumines in their unity the divine quietude and the divine will of action. The ordinary liberation gets the still divine light in the divine quietude, but the integral perfection will aim at this greater triune unity.

When this liberation of the nature comes, there is a liberation also of all the spiritual sense of the dualities of Nature. In the lower nature the dualities are the inevitable effect of the play of the gunas on the soul affected by the formations of the sattwic, rajasic and tamasic ego. The knot of this duality is an ignorance which is unable to seize on the spiritual truth of things and concentrates on the imperfect appearances, but meets them not with a mastery of their inner truth, but with a strife and a shifting balance of attraction and repulsion, capacity and incapacity, liking and disliking, pleasure and pain, joy and sorrow, acceptance and repugnance; all life is represented to us as a tangle of these things, of the pleasant and the unpleasant, the beautiful and the unbeautiful, truth and falsehood, fortune and misfortune, success and failure, good and evil, the inextricable double web of Nature. Attachment to its likings and repugnances keeps the soul bound in this web of good and evil, joys and sorrows. The seeker of liberation gets rid of attachment, throws away from his soul the dualities, but as the dualities appear to be the whole act, stuff and frame of life, this release would seem to be most easily compassed by a withdrawal from life, whether a physical withdrawal, so far as that is possible while in the body, or an inner retirement, a refusal of sanction, a liberating distaste, *vairāgya*, for the whole action of Nature. There is a separation of the soul from Nature. Then the soul watches seated above and unmoved, *udāsīna*, the strife of the gunas in the natural being and regards as an impassive witness the pleasure and pain of the mind and body. Or it is able to impose its indifference even on the outer mind and watches with the impartial calm or the impartial joy of the detached spectator the universal action in which it has no longer an active inner participation. The end of this movement is the rejection of birth and a departure into the silent self, *mokṣa*.

But this rejection is not the last possible word of liberation. The integral liberation comes when this passion for release, *mumukṣutva*, founded on distaste or *vairāgya*, is itself transcended; the soul is then liberated both from attachment to the lower action of nature and from all repugnance to the cosmic action of the Divine. This liberation gets its completeness when the spiritual gnosis can act with a supramental knowledge and reception of the action of Nature and a supramental luminous will in initiation. The gnosis discovers the spiritual sense in Nature, God in things, the soul of good in all things that have the contrary appearance; that soul is delivered in them and out of them, the perversions of the imperfect or contrary forms fall away or are transformed into their higher divine truth,—even as the gunas go back to their divine principles,—and the spirit lives in a universal, infinite and absolute Truth, Good, Beauty, Bliss which is the supramental or ideal divine Nature. The liberation of the Nature becomes one with the liberation of the spirit, and there is founded in the integral freedom the integral perfection.

---

1. This subject has been treated in the Yoga of Works. It is restated here from the point of view of the general type of nature and the complete liberation of the being.

# THE ELEMENTS OF PERFECTION

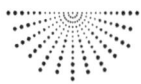

WHEN the self is purified of the wrong and confused action of the instrumental Nature and liberated into its self-existent being, consciousness, power and bliss and the Nature itself liberated from the tangle of this lower action of the struggling gunas and the dualities into the high truth of the divine calm and the divine action, then spiritual perfection becomes possible. Purification and freedom are the indispensable antecedents of perfection. A spiritual self-perfection can only mean a growing into oneness with the nature of divine being, and therefore according to our conception of divine being will be the aim, effort and method of our seeking after this perfection. To the Mayavadin the highest or rather the only real truth of being is the impassive, impersonal, self-aware Absolute and therefore to grow into an impassive calm, impersonality and pure self-awareness of spirit is his idea of perfection and a rejection of cosmic and individual being and a settling into silent self-knowledge is his way. To the Buddhist for whom the highest truth is a negation of being, a recognition of the impermanence and sorrow of being and the disastrous nullity of desire and a dissolution of egoism, of the upholding associations of the Idea and the successions of Karma are the perfect way. Other ideas of the Highest are less negative; each according to its own idea leads towards some likeness to the Divine, *sādṛśya*, and each finds its own way, such as the love and worship of the Bhakta and the growing into the likeness of the Divine by love. But for the integral Yoga perfection will mean a divine spirit and a divine nature which will admit of a divine relation and action in the world; it will mean also in its entirety a divinising of the whole nature, a rejection of all its wrong knots of being and action, but no rejection of any part of our being or of any field of our action. The approach to perfection must be therefore a large and complex movement and its results and workings will have an infinite and varied scope. We must fix in order to find a clue and method on certain essential and fundamental elements and requisites of perfection, *siddhi*; for if these are secured, all the rest will be found to be only their natural development or particular working. We may cast these elements into six divisions, interdependent on each other to a great extent but still in a certain way naturally successive in their order of attainment. The movement will start from a basic equality of the soul and mount to an ideal action of the Divine through our perfected being in the largeness of the Brahmic unity.

The first necessity is some fundamental poise of the soul both in its essential and its natural being regarding and meeting the things, impacts and workings of Nature. This poise we shall arrive at by growing into a perfect equality, *samatā*. The self, spirit or Brahman is one in all and therefore one to all; it is, as is said in the Gita which has developed fully this idea of equality and indicated its experience on at least one side of equality, the equal Brahman, *samaṁ brahma*; the Gita even goes so far in one passage as to identify equality and yoga, *samatvaṁ yoga ucyate*. That is to say, equality is the sign of unity with the Brahman, of becoming Brahman, of growing into an undisturbed spiritual poise of being in the Infinite. Its importance can hardly be exaggerated; for it is the sign of our having passed beyond the egoistic determinations of our nature, of our having conquered our enslaved response to the dualities, of our having transcended the shifting turmoil of the gunas, of our having entered into the calm and peace of liberation. Equality is a term of consciousness which brings into the whole of our being and nature the eternal tranquillity of the Infinite. Moreover, it is the condition of a securely and perfectly divine action; the security and largeness of the cosmic action of the Infinite is based upon and never breaks down or forfeits its eternal tranquillity. That too must be the character of the perfect spiritual action; to be equal and one to all things in spirit, understanding, mind, heart and natural consciousness,—even in the most physical consciousness,— and to make all their workings, whatever their outward adaptation to the thing to be done, always and imminuably full of the divine equality and calm must be its inmost principle. That may be said to be the passive or basic, the fundamental and receptive side of equality, but there is also an active and possessive side, an equal bliss which can only come when the peace of equality is founded and which is the beatific flower of its fullness.

The next necessity of perfection is to raise all the active parts of the human nature to that highest condition and working pitch of their power and capacity, *śakti*, at which they become capable of being divinised into true instruments of the free, perfect, spiritual and divine action. For practical purposes we may take the understanding, the heart, the prana and the body as the four members of our nature which have thus to be prepared, and we have to find the constituent terms of their perfection. Also there is the dynamical force in us (*vīrya*) of the temperament, character and soul nature, *svabhāva*, which makes the power of our members effective in action and gives them their type and direction; this has to be freed from its limitations, enlarged, rounded so that the whole manhood in us may become the basis of a divine manhood, when the Purusha, the real Man in us, the divine Soul, shall act fully in this human instrument and shine fully through this human vessel. To divinise the perfected nature we have to call in the divine Power or Shakti to replace our limited human energy so that this may be shaped into the image of and filled with the force of a greater infinite energy, *daivī prakṛti, bhāgavatī śakti*. This perfection will grow in the measure in which we can surrender ourselves, first, to the guidance and then to the direct action of that Power and of the Master of our being and our works to whom it belongs, and for this purpose faith is the essential, faith is the great motor-power of our being in our aspirations to perfection,—here, a faith in God and the Shakti which shall begin in the heart and understanding, but shall take possession of all our nature, all its consciousness, all its dynamic motive-force. These four things are the essentials of this second element of perfection, the full powers of the members of the instrumental nature, the perfected dynamis of the soul nature, the assumption of them into the action of the divine Power, and a perfect faith in all our members to call and support that assumption, *śakti, vīrya, daivī prakṛti, śraddhā*.

But so long as this development takes place only on the highest level of our normal nature, we may have a reflected and limited image of perfection translated into the lower terms of the soul in mind, life and body, but not the possession of the divine perfection in the highest terms possible to us of the divine Idea and its Power. That is to be found beyond these lower principles in the supramental gnosis; therefore the next step of perfection will be the evolution of the mental into the gnostic being. This evolution is effected by a breaking beyond the mental limitation, a stride upward into the next higher plane or region of our being hidden from us at present by the shining lid of the mental reflections and a conversion of all that we are into the terms of this greater consciousness. In the gnosis itself, *vijñāna*, there are several gradations which open at their highest into the full and infinite Ananda. The gnosis once effectively called into action will progressively take up all the terms of intelligence, will, sense-mind, heart, the vital and sensational being and translate them by a luminous and harmonising conversion into a unity of the truth, power and delight of a divine existence. It will lift into that light and force and convert into their own highest sense our whole intellectual, volitional, dynamic, ethical, aesthetic, sensational, vital and physical being. It has the power also of overcoming physical limitations and developing a more perfect and divinely instrumental body. Its light opens up the fields of the superconscient and darts its rays and pours its luminous flood into the subconscient and enlightens its obscure hints and withheld secrets. It admits us to a greater light of the Infinite than is reflected in the paler luminosity even of the highest mentality. While it perfects the individual soul and nature in the sense of a diviner existence and makes a full harmony of the diversities of our being, it founds all its action upon the Unity from which it proceeds and takes up everything into that Unity. Personality and impersonality, the two eternal aspects of existence, are made one by its action in the spiritual being and Nature body of the Purushottama.

The gnostic perfection, spiritual in its nature, is to be accomplished here in the body and takes life in the physical world as one of its fields, even though the gnosis opens to us possession of planes and worlds beyond the material universe. The physical body is therefore a basis of action, *pratiṣṭhā*, which cannot be despised, neglected or excluded from the spiritual evolution: a perfection of the body as the outer instrument of a complete divine living on earth will be necessarily a part of the gnostic conversion. The change will be effected by bringing in the law of the gnostic Purusha, *vijñānamaya puruṣa*, and of that into which it opens, the Anandamaya, into the physical consciousness and its members. Pushed to its highest conclusion this movement brings in a spiritualising and illumination of the whole physical consciousness and a divinising of the law of the body. For behind the gross physical sheath of this materially visible and sensible frame there is subliminally supporting it and discoverable by a finer subtle consciousness a subtle body of the mental being and a spiritual or causal body of the gnostic and bliss soul in which all the perfection of a spiritual embodiment is to be found, a yet unmanifested divine law of the body. Most of the physical siddhis acquired by certain Yogins are brought about by some opening up of the law of the subtle or a calling down of something of the law of the spiritual body. The ordinary method is the opening up of the *cakras* by the physical processes of Hatha-yoga (of which something is also included in the Raja-yoga) or by the methods of the Tantric discipline. But while these may be optionally used at certain stages by the integral Yoga, they are not indispensable; for here the reliance is on the power of the higher being to change the lower existence, a working is chosen mainly from above downward and not the opposite way, and therefore the development of the superior power of the gnosis will be awaited as the instrumentative change in this part of the Yoga.

There will remain, because it will then only be entirely possible, the perfect action and enjoyment of being on the gnostic basis. The Purusha enters into cosmic manifestation for the variations of his infinite existence, for knowledge, action and enjoyment; the gnosis brings the fullness of spiritual knowledge and it will found on that the divine action and cast the enjoyment of world and being into the law of the truth, the freedom and the perfection of the spirit. But neither action nor enjoyment will be the lower action of the gunas and consequent egoistic enjoyment mostly of the satisfaction of rajasic desire which is our present way of living. Whatever desire will remain, if that name be given, will be the divine desire, the will to delight of the Purusha enjoying in his freedom and perfection the action of the perfected Prakriti and all her members. The Prakriti will take up the whole nature into the law of her higher divine truth and act in that law offering up the universal enjoyment of her action and being to the Anandamaya Ishwara, the Lord of existence and works and Spirit of bliss, who presides over and governs her workings. The individual soul will be the channel of this action and offering, and it will enjoy at once its oneness with the Ishwara and its oneness with the Prakriti and will enjoy all relations with Infinite and finite, with God and the universe and beings in the universe in the highest terms of the union of the universal Purusha and Prakriti.

All the gnostic evolution opens up into the divine principle of Ananda, which is the foundation of the fullness of spiritual being, consciousness and bliss of Sachchidananda or eternal Brahman. Possessed at first by reflection in the mental experience, it will be possessed afterwards with a greater fullness and directness in the massed and luminous consciousness, *cidghana*, which comes by the gnosis. The Siddha or perfected soul will live in union with the Purushottama in this Brahmic consciousness, he will be conscious in the Brahman that is the All, *sarvaṁ brahma*, in the Brahman infinite in being and infinite in quality, *anantaṁ brahma*, in Brahman as self-existent consciousness and universal knowledge, *jñānaṁ brahma*, in Brahman as the self-existent bliss and its universal delight of being, *ānandaṁ brahma*. He will experience all the universe as the manifestation of the One, all quality and action as the play of his universal and infinite energy, all knowledge and conscious experience as the outflowing of that consciousness, and all in the terms of that one Ananda. His physical being will be one with all material Nature, his vital being with the life of the universe, his mind with the cosmic mind, his spiritual knowledge and will with the divine knowledge and will both in itself and as it pours itself through these channels, his spirit with the one spirit in all beings. All the variety of cosmic existence will be changed to him in that unity and revealed in the secret of its spiritual significance. For in this spiritual bliss and being he will be one with That which is the origin and continent and inhabitant and spirit and constituting power of all existence. This will be the highest reach of self-perfection.

# THE PERFECTION OF EQUALITY

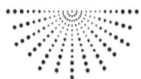

THE VERY first necessity for spiritual perfection is a perfect equality. Perfection in the sense in which we use it in Yoga, means a growth out of a lower undivine into a higher divine nature. In terms of knowledge it is a putting on the being of the higher self and a casting away of the darker broken lower self or a transforming of our imperfect state into the rounded luminous fullness of our real and spiritual personality. In terms of devotion and adoration it is a growing into a likeness of the nature or the law of the being of the Divine, to be united with whom we aspire,—for if there is not this likeness, this oneness of the law of the being, unity between that transcending and universal and this individual spirit is not possible. The supreme divine nature is founded on equality. This affirmation is true of it whether we look on the Supreme Being as a pure silent Self and Spirit or as the divine Master of cosmic existence. The pure Self is equal, unmoved, the witness in an impartial peace of all the happenings and relations of cosmic existence. While it is not averse to them,—aversion is not equality, nor, if that were the attitude of the Self to cosmic existence, could the universe come at all into being or proceed upon its cycles,—a detachment, the calm of an equal regard, a superiority to the reactions which trouble and are the disabling weakness of the soul involved in outward nature, are the very substance of the silent Infinite's purity and the condition of its impartial assent and support to the many-sided movement of the universe. But in that power too of the Supreme which governs and develops these motions, the same equality is a basic condition.

The Master of things cannot be affected or troubled by the reactions of things; if he were, he would be subject to them, not master, not free to develop them according to his sovereign will and wisdom and according to the inner truth and necessity of what is behind their relations, but obliged rather to act according to the claim of temporary accident and phenomenon. The truth of all things is in the calm of their depths, not in the shifting inconstant wave form on the surface. The supreme conscious Being in his divine knowledge and will and love governs their evolution —to our ignorance so often a cruel confusion and distraction—from these depths and is not troubled by the clamour of the surface. The divine nature does not share in our gropings and our passions; when we speak of the divine wrath or favour or of God suffering in man, we are using a human language which mistranslates the inner significance of the movement we characterise. We see something of the real truth of them when we rise out of the phenomenal mind into the heights of the spiritual being. For then we perceive that whether in the silence of self or in its action in the cosmos, the Divine is always Sachchidananda, an infinite existence, an infinite consciousness and self-founded power of conscious being, an infinite bliss in all his existence. We ourselves begin to dwell in an equal light, strength, joy—the psychological rendering of the divine knowledge, will and delight in self and things which are the active universal outpourings from those infinite sources. In the strength of that light, power and joy a secret self and spirit within us accepts and transforms always into food of its perfect experience the dual letters of the mind's transcript of life, and if there were not the hidden greater existence even now within us, we could not bear the pressure of the universal force or subsist in this great and dangerous world. A perfect equality of our spirit and nature is a means by which we can move back from the troubled and ignorant outer consciousness into this inner kingdom of heaven and possess the spirit's eternal kingdoms, *rājyaṁ samṛddham*, of greatness, joy and peace. That self-elevation to the divine nature is the complete fruit and the whole occasion of the discipline of equality demanded from us by the self-perfecting aim in Yoga.

A perfect equality and peace of the soul is indispensable to change the whole substance of our being into substance of the self out of its present stuff of troubled mentality. It is equally indispensable if we aspire to replace our present confused and ignorant action by the self-possessed and luminous works of a free spirit governing its nature and in tune with universal being. A divine action or even a perfect human action is impossible if we have not equality of spirit and an equality in the motive-forces of our nature. The Divine is equal to all, an impartial sustainer of his universe, who views all with equal eyes, assents to the law of developing being which he has brought out of the depths of his existence, tolerates what has to be tolerated, depresses what has to be depressed, raises what has to be raised, creates, sustains and destroys with a perfect and equal understanding of all causes and results and working out of the spiritual and pragmatic meaning of all phenomena. God does not create in obedience to any troubled passion of desire or maintain and preserve through an attachment of partial preference or destroy in a fury of wrath, disgust or aversion. The Divine deals with great and small, just and unjust, ignorant and wise as the Self of all who, deeply intimate and one with the being, leads all according to their nature and need with a perfect understanding, power and justness of proportion. But through it all he moves things according to his large aim in the cycles and draws the soul upward in the evolution through its apparent progress and retrogression towards the higher and ever higher development which is the sense of the cosmic urge. The self-perfecting individual who seeks to be one in will with the Divine and make his nature an instrument of the divine purpose, must enlarge himself out of the egoistic and partial views and motives of the human ignorance and mould himself into an image of this supreme equality.

This equal poise in action is especially necessary for the sadhaka of the integral Yoga. First, he must acquire that equal assent and understanding which will respond to the law of the divine action without trying to impose on it a partial will and the violent claim of a personal aspiration. A wise impersonality, a quiescent equality, a universality which sees all things as the manifestations of the Divine, the one Existence, is not angry, troubled, impatient with the way of things or on the other hand excited, over-eager and precipitate, but sees that the law must be obeyed and the pace of time respected, observes and understands with sympathy the actuality of things and beings, but looks also behind the present appearance to their inner significances and forward to the unrolling of their divine possibilities, is the first thing demanded of those who would do works as the perfect instruments of the Divine. But this impersonal acquiescence is only the basis. Man is the instrument of an evolution which wears at first the mask of a struggle, but grows more and more into its truer and deeper sense of a constant wise adjustment and must take on in a rising scale the deepest truth and significance—now only underlying the adjustment and struggle—of a universal harmony. The perfected human soul must always be an instrument for the hastening of the ways of this evolution. For that a divine power acting with the royalty of the divine will in it must be in whatever degree present in the nature. But to be accomplished and permanent, steadfast in action, truly divine, it has to proceed on the basis of a spiritual equality, a calm, impersonal and equal self-identification with all beings, an understanding of all energies. The Divine acts with a mighty power in the myriad workings of the universe, but with the supporting light and force of an imperturbable oneness, freedom and peace. That must be the type of the perfected soul's divine works. And equality is the condition of the being which makes possible this changed spirit in the action.

But even a human perfection cannot dispense with equality as one of its chief elements and even its essential atmosphere. The aim of a human perfection must include, if it is to deserve the name, two things, self-mastery and a mastery of the surroundings; it must seek for them in the greatest degree of these powers which is at all attainable by our human nature. Man's urge of self-perfection is to be, in the ancient language, *svarāṭ* and *samrāṭ*, self-ruler and king. But to be self-ruler is not possible for him if he is subject to the attack of the lower nature, to the turbulence of grief and joy, to the violent touches of pleasure and pain, to the tumult of his emotions and passions, to the bondage of his personal likings and dislikings, to the strong chains of desire and attachment, to the narrowness of a personal and emotionally preferential judgment and opinion, to all the hundred touches of his egoism and its pursuing stamp on his thought, feeling and action. All these things are the slavery to the lower self which the greater "I" in man must put under his feet if he is to be king of his own nature. To surmount them is the condition of self-rule; but of that surmounting again equality is the condition and the essence of the movement. To be quite free from all these things,—if possible, or at least to be master of and superior to them,—is equality. Farther, one who is not self-ruler, cannot be master of his surroundings. The knowledge, the will, the harmony which is necessary for this outward mastery, can come only as a crown of the inward conquest. It belongs to the self-possessing soul and mind which follows with a disinterested equality the Truth, the Right, the universal Largeness to which alone this mastery is possible,—following always the great ideal they present to our imperfection while it understands and makes a full allowance too for all that seems to conflict with them and stand in the way of their manifestation. This rule is true even on the levels of our actual human mentality, where we can only get a limited perfection. But the ideal of Yoga takes up this aim of Swarajya and Samrajya and puts it on the larger spiritual basis. There it gets its full power, opens to the diviner degrees of the spirit; for it is by oneness with the Infinite, by a spiritual power acting upon finite things, that some highest integral perfection of our being and nature finds its own native foundation.

A perfect equality not only of the self, but in the nature is a condition of the Yoga of self-perfection. The first obvious step to it will be the conquest of our emotional and vital being, for here are the sources of greatest trouble, the most rampant forces of inequality and subjection, the most insistent claim of our imperfection. The equality of these parts of our nature comes by purification and freedom. We might say that equality is the very sign of liberation. To be free from the domination of the urge of vital desire and the stormy mastery of the soul by the passions is to have a calm and equal heart and a life-principle governed by the large and even view of a universal spirit. Desire is the impurity of the Prana, the life-principle, and its chain of bondage. A free Prana means a content and satisfied life-soul which fronts the contact of outward things without desire and receives them with an equal response; delivered, uplifted above the servile duality of liking and disliking, indifferent to the urgings of pleasure and pain, not excited by the pleasant, not troubled and overpowered by the unpleasant, not clinging with attachment to the touches it prefers or violently repelling those for which it has an aversion, it will be opened to a greater system of values of experience. All that comes to it from the world with menace or with solicitation, it will refer to the higher principles, to a reason and heart in touch with or changed by the light and calm joy of the spirit. Thus quieted, mastered by the spirit and no longer trying to impose its own mastery on the deeper and finer soul in us, this life-soul will be itself spiritualised and work as a clear and noble instrument of the diviner dealings of the spirit with things. There is no question here of an ascetic killing of the life-impulse and its native utilities and functions; not its killing is demanded, but its transformation. The function of the Prana is enjoyment, but the real enjoyment of existence is an inward spiritual Ananda, not partial and troubled like that of our vital, emotional or mental pleasure, degraded as they are now by the predominance of the physical mind, but universal, profound, a massed concentration of spiritual bliss possessed in a calm ecstasy of self and all existence. Possession is its function, by possession comes the soul's enjoyment of things, but this is the real possession, a thing large and inward, not dependent on the outward seizing which makes us subject to what we seize. All outward possession and enjoyment will be only an occasion of a satisfied and equal play of the spiritual Ananda with the forms and phenomena of its own world-being. The egoistic possession, the making things our own in the sense of the ego's claim on God and beings and the world, *parigraha*, must be renounced in order that this greater thing, this large, universal and perfect life, may come. *Tyaktena bhuñjīthāḥ*, by renouncing the egoistic sense of desire and possession, the soul enjoys divinely its self and the universe.

A free heart is similarly a heart delivered from the gusts and storms of the affections and the passions; the assailing touch of grief, wrath, hatred, fear, inequality of love, trouble of joy, pain of sorrow fall away from the equal heart, and leave it a thing large, calm, equal, luminous, divine. These things are not incumbent on the essential nature of our being, but the creations of the present make of our outward active mental and vital nature and its transactions with its surroundings. The ego-sense which induces us to act as separate beings who make their isolated claim and experience the test of the values of the universe, is responsible for these aberrations. When we live in unity with the Divine in ourselves and the spirit of the universe, these imperfections fall away from us and disappear in the calm and equal strength and delight of the inner spiritual existence. Always that is within us and transforms the outward touches before they reach it by a passage through a subliminal psychic soul in us which is the hidden instrument of its delight of being. By equality of the heart we get away from the troubled desire-soul on the surface, open the gates of this profounder being, bring out its responses and impose their true divine values on all that solicits our emotional being. A free, happy, equal and all-embracing heart of spiritual feeling is the outcome of this perfection.

In this perfection too there is no question of a severe ascetic insensibility, an aloof spiritual indifference or a strained rugged austerity of self-suppression. This is not a killing of the emotional nature but a transformation. All that presents itself here in our outward nature in perverse or imperfect forms has a significance and utility which come out when we get back to the greater truth of divine being. Love will be not destroyed, but perfected, enlarged to its widest capacity, deepened to its spiritual rapture, the love of God, the love of man, the love of all things as ourselves and as beings and powers of the Divine; a large, universal love, not at all incapable of various relation, will replace the clamant, egoistic, self-regarding love of little joys and griefs and insistent demands afflicted with all the chequered pattern of angers and jealousies and satisfactions, rushings to unity and movements of fatigue, divorce and separation on which we now place so high a value. Grief will cease to exist, but a universal, an equal love and sympathy will take its place, not a suffering sympathy, but a power which, itself delivered, is strong to sustain, to help, to liberate. To the free spirit wrath and hatred are impossible, but not the strong Rudra energy of the Divine which can battle without hatred and destroy without wrath because all the time aware of the things it destroys as parts of itself, its own manifestations and unaltered therefore in its sympathy and understanding of those in whom are embodied these manifestations. All our emotional nature will undergo this high liberating transformation; but in order that it may do so, a perfect equality is the effective condition.

The same equality must be brought into the rest of our being. Our whole dynamic being is acting under the influence of unequal impulses, the manifestations of the lower ignorant nature. These urgings we obey or partially control or place on them the changing and modifying influence of our reason, our refining aesthetic sense and mind and regulating ethical notions. A tangled strain of right and wrong, of useful and harmful, harmonious or disordered activity is the mixed result of our endeavour, a shifting standard of human reason and unreason, virtue and vice, honour and dishonour, the noble and the ignoble, things approved and things disapproved of men, much trouble of self-approbation and disapprobation or of self-righteousness and disgust, remorse, shame and moral depression. These things are no doubt very necessary at present for our spiritual evolution. But the seeker of a greater perfection will draw back from all these dualities, regard them with an equal eye and arrive through equality at an impartial and universal action of the dynamic Tapas, spiritual force, in which his own force and will are turned into pure and just instruments of a greater calm secret of divine working. The ordinary mental standards will be exceeded on the basis of this dynamic equality. The eye of his will must look beyond to a purity of divine being, a motive of divine will-power guided by divine knowledge of which his perfected nature will be the engine, *yantra*. That must remain impossible in entirety as long as the dynamic ego with its subservience to the emotional and vital impulses and the preferences of the personal judgment interferes in his action. A perfect equality of the will is the power which dissolves these knots of the lower impulsion to works. This equality will not respond to the lower impulses, but watch for a greater seeing impulsion from the Light above the mind, and will not judge and govern with the intellectual judgment, but wait for enlightenment and direction from a superior plane of vision. As it mounts upward to the supramental being and widens inward to the spiritual largeness, the dynamic nature will be transformed, spiritualised like the emotional and pranic, and grow into a power of the divine nature. There will be plenty of stumblings and errors and imperfections of adjustment of the instruments to their new working, but the increasingly equal soul will not be troubled overmuch or grieve at these things, since, delivered to the guidance of the Light and Power within self and above mind, it will proceed on its way with a firm assurance and await with growing calm the vicissitudes and completion of the process of transformation. The promise of the Divine Being in the Gita will be the anchor of its resolution, "Abandon all dharmas and take refuge in Me alone; I will deliver thee from all sin and evil; do not grieve."

The equality of the thinking mind will be a part and a very important part of the perfection of the instruments in the nature. Our present attractive self-justifying attachment to our intellectual preferences, our judgments, opinions, imaginations, limiting associations of the memory which makes the basis of our mentality, to the current repetitions of our habitual mind, to the insistences of our pragmatic mind, to the limitations even of our intellectual truth-mind, must go the way of other attachments and yield to the impartiality of an equal vision. The equal thought-mind will look on knowledge and ignorance and on truth and error, those dualities created by our limited nature of consciousness and the partiality of our intellect and its little stock of reasonings and intuitions, accept them both without being bound to either twine of the skein and await a luminous transcendence. In ignorance it will see a knowledge which is imprisoned and seeks or waits for delivery, in error a truth at work which has lost itself or got thrown by the groping mind into misleading forms. On the other side it will not hold itself bound and limited by its knowledge or forbidden by it to proceed to fresh illumination, nor lay too fierce a grasp on truth, even when using it to the full, or tyrannously chain it to its present formulations. This perfect equality of the thinking mind is indispensable because the objective of this progress is the greater light which belongs to a higher plane of spiritual cognizance. This equality is the most delicate and difficult of all, the least practised by the human mind; its perfection is impossible so long as the supramental light does not fall fully on the upward looking mentality. But an increasing will to equality in the intelligence is needed, before that light can work freely upon the mental substance. This too is not an abnegation of the seekings and cosmic purposes of the intelligence, not an indifference or impartial scepticism, nor yet a stilling of all thought in the silence of the Ineffable. A stilling of the mental thought may be part of the discipline, when the object is to free the mind from its own partial workings, in order that it may become an equal channel of a higher light and knowledge; but there must also be a transformation of the mental substance; otherwise the higher light cannot assume full possession and a compelling shape for the ordered works of the divine consciousness in the human being. The silence of the Ineffable is a truth of divine being, but the Word which proceeds from that silence is also a truth, and it is this Word which has to be given a body in the conscious form of the nature.

But, finally, all this equalisation of the nature is a preparation for the highest spiritual equality to take possession of the whole being and make a pervading atmosphere in which the light, power and joy of the Divine can manifest itself in man amid an increasing fullness. That equality is the eternal equality of Sachchidananda. It is an equality of the infinite being which is self-existent, an equality of the eternal spirit, but it will mould into its own mould the mind, heart, will, life, physical being. It is an equality of the infinite spiritual consciousness which will contain and base the blissful flowing and satisfied waves of a divine knowledge. It is an equality of the divine Tapas which will initiate a luminous action of the divine will in all the nature. It is an equality of the divine Ananda which will found the play of a divine universal delight, universal love and an illimitable aesthesis of universal beauty. The ideal equal peace and calm of the Infinite will be the wide ether of our perfected being, but the ideal, equal and perfect action of the Infinite through the nature working on the relations of the universe will be the untroubled outpouring of its power in our being. This is the meaning of equality in the terms of the integral Yoga.

# THE WAY OF EQUALITY

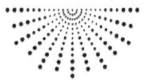

IT WILL appear from the description of the complete and perfect equality that this equality has two sides. It must therefore be arrived at by two successive movements. One will liberate us from the action of the lower nature and admit us to the calm peace of the divine being; the other will liberate us into the full being and power of the higher nature and admit us to the equal poise and universality of a divine and infinite knowledge, will of action, Ananda. The first may be described as a passive or negative equality, an equality of reception which fronts impassively the impacts and phenomena of existence and negates the dualities of the appearances and reactions which they impose on us. The second is an active, a positive equality which accepts the phenomena of existence, but only as the manifestation of the one divine being and with an equal response to them which comes from the divine nature in us and transforms them into its hidden values. The first lives in the peace of the one Brahman and puts away from it the nature of the active Ignorance. The second lives in that peace, but also in the Ananda of the Divine and imposes on the life of the soul in nature the signs of the divine knowledge, power and bliss of being. It is this double orientation united by the common principle which will determine the movement of equality in the integral Yoga.

The effort towards a passive or purely receptive equality may start from three different principles or attitudes which all lead to the same result and ultimate consequence,—endurance, indifference and submission. The principle of endurance relies on the strength of the spirit within us to bear all the contacts, impacts, suggestions of this phenomenal Nature that besieges us on every side without being overborne by them and compelled to bear their emotional, sensational, dynamic, intellectual reactions. The outer mind in the lower nature has not this strength. Its strength is that of a limited force of consciousness which has to do the best it can with all that comes in upon it or besieges it from the greater whirl of consciousness and energy which environs it on this plane of existence. That it can maintain itself at all and affirm its individual being in the universe, is due indeed to the strength of the spirit within it, but it cannot bring forward the whole of that strength or the infinity of that force to meet the attacks of life; if it could, it would be at once the equal and master of its world. In fact, it has to manage as it can. It meets certain impacts and is able to assimilate, equate or master them partially or completely, for a time or wholly, and then it has in that degree the emotional and sensational reactions of joy, pleasure, satisfaction, liking, love, etc., or the intellectual and mental reactions of acceptance, approval, understanding, knowledge, preference, and on these its will seizes with attraction, desire, the attempt to prolong, to repeat, to create, to possess, to make them the pleasurable habit of its life. Other impacts it meets, but finds them too strong for it or too dissimilar and discordant or too weak to give it satisfaction; these are things which it cannot bear or cannot equate with itself or cannot assimilate, and it is obliged to give to them reactions of grief, pain, discomfort, dissatisfaction, disliking, disapproval, rejection, inability to understand or know, refusal of admission. Against them it seeks to protect itself, to escape from them, to avoid or minimise their recurrence; it has with regard to them movements of fear, anger, shrinking, horror, aversion, disgust, shame, would gladly be delivered from them, but it cannot get away from them, for it is bound to and even invites their causes and therefore the results; for these impacts are part of life, tangled up with the things we desire, and the inability to deal with them is part of the imperfection of our nature. Other impacts again the normal mind succeeds in holding at bay or neutralising and to these it has a natural reaction of indifference, insensibility or tolerance which is neither positive acceptance and enjoyment nor rejection or suffering. To things, persons, happenings, ideas, workings, whatever presents itself to the mind, there are always these three kinds of reaction. At the same time, in spite of their generality, there is nothing absolute about them;

they form a scheme for a habitual scale which is not precisely the same for all or even for the same mind at different times or in different conditions. The same impact may arouse in it at one time and another the pleasurable or positive, the adverse or negative or the indifferent or neutral reactions.

The soul which seeks mastery may begin by turning upon these reactions the encountering and opposing force of a strong and equal endurance. Instead of seeking to protect itself from or to shun and escape the unpleasant impacts it may confront them and teach itself to suffer and to bear them with perseverance, with fortitude, an increasing equanimity or an austere or calm acceptance. This attitude, this discipline brings out three results, three powers of the soul in relation to things. First, it is found that what was before unbearable, becomes easy to endure; the scale of the power that meets the impact rises in degree; it needs a greater and greater force of it or of its protracted incidence to cause trouble, pain, grief, aversion or any other of the notes in the gamut of the unpleasant reactions. Secondly, it is found that the conscious nature divides itself into two parts, one of the normal mental and emotional nature in which the customary reactions continue to take place, another of the higher will and reason which observes and is not troubled or affected by the passion of this lower nature, does not accept it as its own, does not approve, sanction or participate. Then the lower nature begins to lose the force and power of its reactions, to submit to the suggestions of calm and strength from the higher reason and will, and gradually that calm and strength take possession of the mental and emotional, even of the sensational, vital and physical being. This brings the third power and result, the power by this endurance and mastery, this separation and rejection of the lower nature, to get rid of the normal reactions and even, if we will, to remould all our modes of experience by the strength of the spirit. This method is applied not only to the unpleasant, but also to the pleasant reactions; the soul refuses to give itself up to or be carried away by them; it endures with calm the impacts which bring joy and pleasure; refuses to be excited by them and replaces the joy and eager seeking of the mind after pleasant things by the calm of the spirit. It can be applied too to the thought-mind in a calm reception of knowledge and of limitation of knowledge which refuses to be carried away by the fascination of this attractive or repelled by dislike for that unaccustomed or unpalatable thought-suggestion and waits on the Truth with a detached observation which allows it to grow on the strong, disinterested, mastering will and reason. Thus the soul becomes gradually equal to all things, master of itself, adequate to meet the world with a strong front in the mind and an undisturbed serenity of the spirit.

The second way is an attitude of impartial indifference. Its method is to reject at once the attraction or the repulsion of things, to cultivate for them a luminous impassivity, an inhibiting rejection, a habit of dissociation and desuetude. This attitude reposes less on the will, though will is always necessary, than on the knowledge. It is an attitude which regards these passions of the mind as things born of the illusion of the outward mentality or inferior movements unworthy of the calm truth of the single and equal spirit or a vital and emotional disturbance to be rejected by the tranquil observing will and dispassionate intelligence of the sage. It puts away desire from the mind, discards the ego which attributes these dual values to things, and replaces desire by an impartial and indifferent peace and ego by the pure self which is not troubled, excited or unhinged by the impacts of the world. And not only is the emotional mind quieted, but the intellectual being also rejects the thoughts of the ignorance and rises beyond the interests of an inferior knowledge to the one truth that is eternal and without change. This way too develops three results or powers by which it ascends to peace.

First, it is found that the mind is voluntarily bound by the petty joys and troubles of life and that in reality these can have no inner hold on it, if the soul simply chooses to cast off its habit of helpless determination by external and transient things. Secondly, it is found that here too a division can be made, a psychological partition between the lower or outward mind still subservient to the old habitual touches and the higher reason and will which stand back to live in the indifferent calm of the spirit. There grows on us, in other words, an inner separate calm which watches the commotion of the lower members without taking part in it or giving it any sanction. At first the higher reason and will may be often clouded, invaded, the mind carried away by the incitation of the lower members, but eventually this calm becomes inexpugnable, permanent, not to be shaken by the most violent touches, *na duḥkhena guruṇāpi vicālyate*. This inner soul of calm regards the trouble of the outer mind with a detached superiority or a passing uninvolved indulgence such as might be given to the trivial joys and griefs of a child, it does not regard them as its own or as reposing on any permanent reality. And, finally, the outer mind too accepts by degrees this calm and indifferent serenity; it ceases to be attracted by the things that attracted it or troubled by the griefs and pains to which it had the habit of attaching an unreal importance. Thus the third power comes, an all-pervading power of wide tranquillity and peace, a bliss of release from the siege of our imposed fantastic self-torturing nature, the deep undisturbed exceeding happiness of the touch of the eternal and infinite replacing by its permanence the strife and turmoil of impermanent things, *brahmasaṁsparśam atyantaṁ sukham aśnute*. The soul is fixed in the delight of the self, *ātmaratiḥ*, in the single and infinite Ananda of the spirit and hunts no more after outward touches and their griefs and pleasures. It observes the world only as the spectator of a play or action in which it is no longer compelled to participate.

The third way is that of submission, which may be the Christian resignation founded on submission to the will of God, or an unegoistic acceptance of things and happenings as a manifestation of the universal Will in time, or a complete surrender of the person to the Divine, to the supreme Purusha. As the first was a way of the will and the second a way of knowledge, of the understanding reason, so this is a way of the temperament and heart and very intimately connected with the principle of Bhakti. If it is pushed to the end, it arrives at the same result of a perfect equality. For the knot of the ego is loosened and the personal claim begins to disappear, we find that we are no longer bound to joy in things pleasant or sorrow over the unpleasant; we bear them without either eager acceptance or troubled rejection, refer them to the Master of our being, concern ourselves less and less with their personal result to us and hold only one thing of importance, to approach God, or to be in touch and tune with the universal and infinite Existence, or to be united with the Divine, his channel, instrument, servant, lover, rejoicing in him and in our relation with him and having no other object or cause of joy or sorrow. Here too there may be for some time a division between the lower mind of habitual emotions and the higher psychical mind of love and self-giving, but eventually the former yields, changes, transforms itself, is swallowed up in the love, joy, delight of the Divine and has no other interests or attractions. Then all within is the equal peace and bliss of that union, the one silent bliss that passes understanding, the peace that abides untouched by the solicitation of lower things in the depths of our spiritual existence.

These three ways coincide in spite of their separate starting points, first, by their inhibition of the normal reactions of the mind to the touches of outward things, *bāhya-sparśān*, secondly, by their separation of the self or spirit from the outward action of Nature. But it is evident that our perfection will be greater and more embracingly complete, if we can have a more active equality which will enable us not only to draw back from or confront the world in a detached and separated calm, but to return upon it and possess it in the power of the calm and equal Spirit. This is possible because the world, Nature, action are not in fact a quite separate thing, but a manifestation of the Self, the All-Soul, the Divine. The reactions of the normal mind are a degradation of the divine values which would but for this degradation make this truth evident to us,—a falsification, an ignorance which alters their workings, an ignorance which starts from the involution of the Self in a blind material nescience. Once we return to the full consciousness of Self, of God, we can then put a true divine value on things and receive and act on them with the calm, joy, knowledge, seeing will of the Spirit. When we begin to do that, then the soul begins to have an equal joy in the universe, an equal will dealing with all energies, an equal knowledge which takes possession of the spiritual truth behind all the phenomena of this divine manifestation. It possesses the world as the Divine possesses it, in a fullness of the infinite light, power and Ananda.

All this existence can therefore be approached by a Yoga of positive and active in place of the negative and passive equality. This requires, first, a new knowledge which is the knowledge of unity,—to see all things as oneself and to see all things in God and God in all things. There is then a will of equal acceptance of all phenomena, all events, all happenings, all persons and forces as masks of the Self, movements of the one energy, results of the one power in action, ruled by the one divine wisdom; and on the foundation of this will of greater knowledge there grows a strength to meet everything with an untroubled soul and mind. There must be an idendification of myself with the self of the universe, a vision and a feeling of oneness with all creatures, a perception of all forces and energies and results as the movement of this energy of my self and therefore intimately my own; not, obviously, of my ego-self which must be silenced, eliminated, cast away,—otherwise this perfection cannot come,—but of a greater impersonal or universal self with which I am now one. For my personality is now only one centre of action of that universal self, but a centre intimately in relation and unison with all other personalities and also with all those other things which are to us only impersonal objects and forces: but in fact they also are powers of the one impersonal Person (Purusha), God, Self and Spirit. My individuality is his and is no longer a thing incompatible with or separated from universal being; it is itself universalised, a knower of the universal Ananda and one with and a lover of all that it knows, acts on and enjoys. For to the equal knowledge of the universe and equal will of acceptance of the universe will be added an equal delight in all the cosmic manifestation of the Divine.

Here too we may describe three results or powers of the method. First, we develop this power of equal acceptance in the spirit and in the higher reason and will which respond to the spiritual knowledge. But also we find that though the nature can be induced to take this general attitude, there is yet a struggle between that higher reason and will and the lower mental being which clings to the old egoistic way of seeing the world and reacting to its impacts. Then we find that these two, though at first confused, mingled together, alternating, acting on each other, striving for possession, can be divided, the higher spiritual disengaged from the lower mental nature. But in this stage, while the mind is still subject to reactions of grief, trouble, an inferior joy and pleasure, there is an increased difficulty which does not act to the same extent in a more sharply individualised Yoga. For not only does the mind feel its own troubles and difficulties, but it shares in the joys and griefs of others, vibrates to them in a poignant sympathy, feels their impacts with a subtle sensitiveness, makes them its own; not only so, but the difficulties of others are added to our own and the forces which oppose the perfection act with a greater persistence, because they feel this movement to be an attack upon and an attempt to conquer their universal kingdom and not merely the escape of an isolated soul from their empire. But finally, we find too that there comes a power to surmount these difficulties; the higher reason and will impose themselves on the lower mind, which sensibly changes into the vast types of the spiritual nature; it takes even a delight in feeling, meeting and surmounting all troubles, obstacles and difficulties until they are eliminated by its own transformation. Then the whole being lives in a final power, the universal calm and joy, the seeing delight and will of the Spirit in itself and its manifestation.

To see how this positive method works, we may note very briefly its principle in the three great powers of knowledge, will and feeling. All emotion, feeling, sensation is a way of the soul meeting and putting effective values on the manifestations of the Self in nature. But what the self feels is a universal delight, Ananda. The soul in the lower mind on the contrary gives it, as we have seen, three varying values of pain, pleasure and neutral indifference, which tone by gradations of less and more into each other, and this gradation depends on the power of the individualised consciousness to meet, sense, assimilate, equate, master all that comes in on it from all of the greater self which it has by separative individualisation put outside of it and made as if not-self to its experience. But all the time, because of the greater Self within us, there is a secret soul which takes delight in all these things and draws strength from and grows by all that touches it, profits as much by adverse as by favourable experience. This can make itself felt by the outer desire soul, and that in fact is why we have a delight in existing and can even take a certain kind of pleasure in struggle, suffering and the harsher colours of existence. But to get the universal Ananda all our instruments must learn to take not any partial or perverse, but the essential joy of all things. In all things there is a principle of Ananda, which the understanding can seize on and the aesthesis feel as the taste of delight in them, their *rasa*; but ordinarily they put upon them instead arbitrary, unequal and contrary values: they have to be led to perceive things in the light of the spirit and to transform these provisional values into the real, the equal and essential, the spiritual *rasa*. The life-principle is there to give this seizing of the principle of delight, *rasa-grahaṇa*, the form of a strong possessing enjoyment, *bhoga*, which makes the whole life-being vibrate with it and accept and rejoice in it; but ordinarily it is not, owing to desire, equal to its task, but turns it into the three lower forms,—pain and pleasure, *sukha-bhoga duḥkha-bhoga*, and that rejection of both which we call insensibility or indifference. The prana or vital being has to be liberated from desire and its inequalities and to accept and turn into pure enjoyment the *rasa* which the understanding and aesthesis perceive. Then there is no farther obstacle in the instruments to the third step by which all is changed into the full and pure ecstasy of the spiritual Ananda.

In the matter of knowledge, there are again three reactions of the mind to things, ignorance, error and true knowledge. The positive equality will accept all three of them to start with as movements of a self-manifestation which evolves out of ignorance through the partial or distorted knowledge which is the cause of error to true knowledge. It will deal with the ignorance of the mind, as what it is psychologically, a clouded, veiled or wrapped-up state of the substance of consciousness in which the knowledge of the all-knowing Self is hidden as if in a dark sheath; it will dwell on it by the mind and by the aid of related truths already known, by the intelligence or by an intuitive concentration deliver the knowledge out of the veil of the ignorance. It will not attach itself only to the known or try to force all into its little frame, but will dwell on the known and the unknown with an equal mind open to all possibility. So too it will deal with error; it will accept the tangled skein of truth and error, but attach itself to no opinion, rather seeking for the element of truth behind all opinions, the knowledge concealed within the error,—for all error is a disfiguration of some misunderstood fragments of truth and draws its vitality from that and not from its misapprehension; it will accept, but not limit itself even by ascertained truths, but will always be ready for new knowledge and seek for a more and more integral, a more and more extended, reconciling, unifying wisdom. This can only come in its fullness by rising to the ideal supermind, and therefore the equal seeker of truth will not be attached to the intellect and its workings or think that all ends there, but be prepared to rise beyond, accepting each stage of ascent and the contributions of each power of his being, but only to lift them into a higher truth. He must accept everything, but cling to nothing, be repelled by nothing however imperfect or however subversive of fixed notions, but also allow nothing to lay hold on him to the detriment of the free working of the Truth-Spirit. This equality of the intelligence is an essential condition for rising to the higher supramental and spiritual knowledge.

The will in us, because it is the most generally forceful power of our being,—there is a will of knowledge, a will of life, a will of emotion, a will acting in every part of our nature,—takes many forms and returns various reactions to things, such as incapacity, limitation of power, mastery, or right will, wrong or perverted will, neutral volition,—in the ethical mind virtue, sin and non-ethical volition,—and others of the kind.

These too the positive equality accepts as a tangle of provisional values from which it must start, but which it must transform into universal mastery, into the will of the Truth and universal Right, into the freedom of the divine Will in action. The equal will need not feel remorse, sorrow or discouragement over its stumblings; if these reactions occur in the habitual mentality, it will only see how far they indicate an imperfection and the thing to be corrected,—for they are not always just indicators,—and so get beyond them to a calm and equal guidance. It will see that these stumblings themselves are necessary to experience and in the end steps towards the goal. Behind and within all that occurs in ourselves and in the world, it will look for the divine meaning and the divine guidance; it will look beyond imposed limitations to the voluntary self-limitation of the universal Power by which it regulates its steps and gradations,—imposed on our ignorance, self-imposed in the divine knowledge,—and go beyond to unity with the illimitable power of the Divine. All energies and actions it will see as forces proceeding from the one Existence and their perversions as imperfections, inevitable in the developing movement, of powers that were needed for that movement; it will therefore have charity for all imperfections, even while pressing steadily towards a universal perfection. This equality will open the nature to the guidance of the divine and universal Will and make it ready for that supramental action in which the power of the soul in us is luminously full of and one with the power of the supreme Spirit.

The integral Yoga will make use of both the passive and the active methods according to the need of the nature and the guidance of the inner spirit, the Antaryamin. It will not limit itself by the passive way, for that would lead only to some individual quietistic salvation or negation of an active and universal spiritual being which would be inconsistent with the totality of its aim. It will use the method of endurance, but not stop short with a detached strength and serenity, but move rather to a positive strength and mastery, in which endurance will no longer be needed, since the self will then be in a calm and powerful spontaneous possession of the universal energy and capable of determining easily and happily all its reactions in the oneness and the Ananda. It will use the method of impartial indifference, but not end in an aloof indifference to all things, but rather move towards a high-seated impartial acceptance of life strong to transform all experience into the greater values of the equal spirit. It will use too temporarily resignation and submission, but by the full surrender of its personal being to the Divine it will attain to the all-possessing Ananda in which there is no need of resignation, to the perfect harmony with the universal which is not merely an acquiescence, but an embracing oneness, to the perfect instrumentality and subjection of the natural self to the Divine by which the Divine also is possessed by the individual spirit. It will use fully the positive method, but will go beyond any individual acceptance of things which would have the effect of turning existence into a field only of the perfected individual knowledge, power and Ananda. That it will have, but also it will have the oneness by which it can live in the existence of others for their sake and not only for its own and for their assistance and as one of their means, an associated and helping force in the movement towards the same perfection. It will live for the Divine, not shunning world-existence, not attached to the earth or the heavens, not attached either to a supracosmic liberation, but equally one with the Divine in all his planes and able to live in him equally in the Self and in the manifestation.

# THE ACTION OF EQUALITY

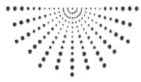

THE DISTINCTIONS that have already been made, will have shown in sufficiency what is meant by the status of equality. It is not mere quiescence and indifference, not a withdrawal from experience, but a superiority to the present reactions of the mind and life. It is the spiritual way of replying to life or rather of embracing it and compelling it to become a perfect form of action of the self and spirit. It is the first secret of the soul's mastery of existence. When we have it in perfection, we are admitted to the very ground of the divine spiritual nature. The mental being in the body tries to compel and conquer life, but is at every turn compelled by it, because it submits to the desire reactions of the vital self. To be equal, not to be overborne by any stress of desire, is the first condition of real mastery, self-empire is its basis. But a mere mental equality, however great it may be, is hampered by the tendency of quiescence. It has to preserve itself from desire by self-limitation in the will and action. It is only the spirit which is capable of sublime undisturbed rapidities of will as well as an illimitable patience, equally just in a slow and deliberate or a swift and violent, equally secure in a safely lined and limited or a vast and enormous action. It can accept the smallest work in the narrowest circle of cosmos, but it can work too upon the whirl of chaos with an understanding and creative force; and these things it can do because by its detached and yet intimate acceptance it carries into both an infinite calm, knowledge, will and power. It has that detachment because it is above all the happenings, forms, ideas and movements it embraces in its scope; and it has that intimate acceptance because it is yet one with all things. If we have not this free unity, *ekatvam anupaśyataḥ*, we have not the full equality of the spirit.

The first business of the sadhaka is to see whether he has the perfect equality, how far he has gone in this direction or else where is the flaw, and to exercise steadily his will on his nature or invite the will of the Purusha to get rid of the defect and its causes. There are four things that he must have; first, equality in the most concrete practical sense of the word, *samatā*, freedom from mental, vital, physical preferences, an even acceptance of all God's workings within and around him; secondly, a firm peace and absence of all disturbance and trouble, *śānti*; thirdly, a positive inner spiritual happiness and spiritual ease of the natural being which nothing can lessen, *sukham*; fourthly, a clear joy and laughter of the soul embracing life and existence. To be equal is to be infinite and universal, not to limit oneself, not to bind oneself down to this or that form of the mind and life and its partial preferences and desires. But since man in his present normal nature lives by his mental and vital formations, not in the freedom of his spirit, attachment to them and the desires and references they involve is also his normal condition. To accept them is at first inevitable, to get beyond them exceedingly difficult and not, perhaps, altogether possible so long as we are compelled to use the mind as the chief instrument of our action. The first necessity therefore is to take at least the sting out of them, to deprive them, even when they persist, of their greater insistence, their present egoism, their more violent claim on our nature.

The test that we have done this is the presence of an undisturbed calm in the mind and spirit. The sadhaka must be on the watch as the witnessing and willing Purusha behind or, better, as soon as he can manage it, above the mind, and repel even the least indices or incidence of trouble, anxiety, grief, revolt, disturbance in his mind. If these things come, he must at once detect their source, the defect which they indicate, the fault of egoistic claim, vital desire, emotion or idea from which they start and this he must discourage by his will, his spiritualised intelligence, his soul unity with the Master of his being. On no account must he admit any excuse for them, however natural, righteous in seeming or plausible, or any inner or outer justification. If it is the prana which is troubled and clamorous, he must separate himself from the troubled prana, keep seated his higher nature in the buddhi and by the buddhi school and reject the claim of the desire-soul in him; and so too if it is the heart of emotion that makes the clamour and the disturbance. If on the other hand it is the will and intelligence itself that is at fault, then the trouble is more difficult to command, because then his chief aid and instrument becomes an accomplice of the revolt against the divine Will and the old sins of the lower members take advantage of this sanction to raise their diminished heads. Therefore there must be a constant insistence on one main idea, the self-surrender to the Master of our being, God within us and in the world, the supreme Self, the universal Spirit. The buddhi dwelling always in this master idea must discourage all its own lesser insistences and preferences and teach the whole being that the ego whether it puts forth its claim through the reason, the personal will, the heart or the desire-soul in the prana, has no just claim of any kind and all grief, revolt, impatience, trouble is a violence against the Master of the being.

This complete self-surrender must be the chief mainstay of the sadhaka because it is the only way, apart from complete quiescence and indifference to all action,—and that has to be avoided,—by which the absolute calm and peace can come. The persistence of trouble, *aśānti*, the length of time taken for this purification and perfection, itself must not be allowed to become a reason for discouragement and impatience. It comes because there is still something in the nature which responds to it, and the recurrence of trouble serves to bring out the presence of the defect, put the sadhaka upon his guard and bring about a more enlightened and consistent action of the will to get rid of it. When the trouble is too strong to be kept out, it must be allowed to pass and its return discouraged by a greater vigilance and insistence of the spiritualised buddhi. Thus persisting, it will be found that these things lose their force more and more, become more and more external and brief in their recurrence, until finally calm becomes the law of the being. This rule persists so long as the mental buddhi is the chief instrument; but when the supramental light takes possession of mind and heart, then there can be no trouble, grief or disturbance; for that brings with it a spiritual nature of illumined strength in which these things can have no place. There the only vibrations and emotions are those which belong to the *ānandamaya* nature of divine unity.

The calm established in the whole being must remain the same whatever happens, in health and disease, in pleasure and in pain, even in the strongest physical pain, in good fortune and misfortune, our own or that of those we love, in success and failure, honour and insult, praise and blame, justice done to us or injustice, everything that ordinarily affects the mind. If we see unity everywhere, if we recognise that all comes by the divine will, see God in all, in our enemies or rather our opponents in the game of life as well as our friends, in the powers that oppose and resist us as well as the powers that favour and assist, in all energies and forces and happenings, and if besides we can feel that all is undivided from our self, all the world one with us within our universal being, then this attitude becomes much easier to the heart and mind. But even before we can attain or are firmly seated in that universal vision, we have by all the means in our power to insist on this receptive and active equality and calm. Even something of it, *alpam api asya dharmasya*, is a great step towards perfection; a first firmness in it is the beginning of liberated perfection; its completeness is the perfect assurance of a rapid progress in all the other members of perfection. For without it we can have no solid basis; and by the pronounced lack of it we shall be constantly falling back to the lower status of desire, ego, duality, ignorance.

This calm once attained, vital and mental preference has lost its disturbing force; it only remains as a formal habit of the mind. Vital acceptance or rejection, the greater readiness to welcome this rather than that happening, the mental acceptance or rejection, the preference of this more congenial to that other less congenial idea or truth, the dwelling upon the will to this rather than to that other result, become a formal mechanism still necessary as an index of the direction in which the Shakti is meant to turn or for the present is made to incline by the Master of our being. But it loses its disturbing aspect of strong egoistic will, intolerant desire, obstinate liking. These appearances may remain for a while in a diminished form, but as the calm of equality increases, deepens, becomes more essential and compact, *ghana*, they disappear, cease to colour the mental and vital substance or occur only as touches on the most external physical mind, are unable to penetrate within, and at last even that recurrence, that appearance at the outer gates of mind ceases. Then there can come the living reality of the perception that all in us is done and directed by the Master of our being, *yathā prayukto 'smi, tathā karomi*, which was before only a strong idea and faith with occasional and derivative glimpses of the divine action behind the becomings of our personal nature. Now every movement is seen to be the form given by the Shakti, the divine power in us, to the indications of the Purusha, still no doubt personalised, still belittled in the inferior mental form, but not primarily egoistic, an imperfect form, not a positive deformation. We have then to get beyond this stage even. For the perfect action and experience is not to be determined by any kind of mental or vital preference, but by the revealing and inspiring spiritual will which is the Shakti in her direct and real initiation. When I say that as I am appointed, I work, I still bring in a limiting personal element and mental reaction. But it is the Master who will do his own work through myself as his instrument, and there must be no mental or other preference in me to limit, to interfere, to be a source of imperfect working. The mind must become a silent luminous channel for the revelations of the supramental Truth and of the Will involved in its seeing. Then shall the action be the action of that highest Being and Truth and not a qualified translation or mistranslation in the mind. Whatever limitation, selection, relation is imposed, will be self-imposed by the Divine on himself in the individual at the moment for his own purpose, not binding, not final, not an ignorant determination of the mind. The thought and will become then an action from a luminous Infinite, a formulation not excluding other formulations, but rather putting them into their just place in relation to itself, englobing or transforming them even and proceeding to larger formations of the divine knowledge and action.

The first calm that comes is of the nature of peace, the absence of all unquiet, grief and disturbance. As the equality becomes more intense, it takes on a fuller substance of positive happiness and spiritual ease. This is the joy of the spirit in itself, dependent on nothing external for its absolute existence, *nirāśraya*, as the Gita describes it, *antaḥ-sukho antarārāmaḥ*, an exceeding inner happiness, *brahmasaṁsparśam atyantaṁ sukham aśnute*. Nothing can disturb it, and it extends itself to the soul's view of outward things, imposes on them too the law of this quiet spiritual joy. For the base of it is still calm, it is an even and tranquil neutral joy, *ahaituka*. And as the supramental light grows, a greater Ananda comes, the base of the abundant ecstasy of the spirit in all it is, becomes, sees, experiences and of the laughter of the Shakti doing luminously the work of the Divine and taking his Ananda in all the worlds.

The perfected action of equality transforms all the values of things on the basis of the divine *ānandamaya* power. The outward action may remain what it was or may change, that must be as the Spirit directs and according to the need of the work to be done for the world,—but the whole inner action is of another kind. The Shakti in its different powers of knowledge, action, enjoyment, creation, formulation, will direct itself to the different aims of existence, but in another spirit; they will be the aims, the fruits, the lines of working laid down by the Divine from his light above, not anything claimed by the ego for its own separate sake. The mind, the heart, the vital being, the body itself will be satisfied with whatever comes to them from the dispensation of the Master of the being and in that find a subtlest and yet fullest spiritualised satisfaction and delight; but the divine knowledge and will above will work forward towards its farther ends. Here both success and failure lose their present meanings. There can be no failure; for whatever happens is the intention of the Master of the worlds, not final, but a step on his way, and if it appears as an opposition, a defeat, a denial, even for the moment a total denial of the aim set before the instrumental being, it is so only in appearance and afterwards it will appear in its right place in the economy of his action,—a fuller supramental vision may even see at once or beforehand its necessity and its true relation to the eventual result to which it seems so contrary and even perhaps its definite prohibition. Or, if—while the light is deficient—there has been a misinterpretation whether with regard to the aim or the course of the action and the steps of the result, the failure comes as a rectification and is calmly accepted without bringing discouragement or a fluctuation of the will. In the end it is found that there is no such thing as failure and the soul takes an equal passive or active delight in all happenings as the steps and formulations of the divine Will. The same evolution takes place with regard to good fortune and ill fortune, the pleasant and the unpleasant in every form, *mangala amangala, priya apriya*.

And as with happenings, so with persons, equality brings an entire change of the view and the attitude. The first result of the equal mind and spirit is to bring about an increasing charity and inner toleration of all persons, ideas, views, actions, because it is seen that God is in all beings and each acts according to his nature, his *svabhāva*, and its present formulations. When there is the positive equal Ananda, this deepens to a sympathetic understanding and in the end an equal universal love. None of these things need prevent various relations or different formulations of the inner attitude according to the need of life as determined by the spiritual will, or firm furtherings of this idea, view, action against that other for the same need and purpose by the same determination, or a strong outward or inward resistance, opposition and action against the forces that are impelled to stand in the way of the decreed movement. And there may be even the rush of the Rudra energy forcefully working upon or shattering the human or other obstacle, because that is necessary both for him and for the world purpose. But the essence of the equal inmost attitude is not altered or diminished by these more superficial formulations. The spirit, the fundamental soul remain the same, even while the Shakti of knowledge, will, action, love does its work and assumes the various forms needed for its work. And in the end all becomes a form of a luminous spiritual unity with all persons, energies, things in the being of God and in the luminous, spiritual, one and universal force, in which one's own action becomes an inseparable part of the action of all, is not divided from it, but feels perfectly every relation as a relation with God in all in the complex terms of his universal oneness. That is a plenitude which can hardly be described in the language of the dividing mental reason for it uses all its oppositions, yet escapes from them, nor can it be put in the terms of our limited mental psychology. It belongs to another domain of consciousness, another plane of our being.

# THE POWER OF THE INSTRUMENTS

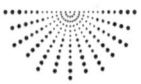

THE SECOND member of the Yoga of self-perfection is the heightened, enlarged and rectified power of the instruments of our normal Nature. The cultivation of this second perfection need not wait for the security of the equal mind and spirit, but it is only in that security that it can become complete and act in the safety of the divine leading. The object of this cultivation is to make the nature a fit instrument for divine works. All work is done by power, by Shakti, and since the integral Yoga does not contemplate abandonment of works, but rather a doing of all works from the divine consciousness and with the supreme guidance, the characteristic powers of the instruments, mind, life and body, must not only be purified of defects, but raised to a capacity for this greater action. In the end they must undergo a spiritual and supramental transfiguration.

There are four members of this second part of the sadhana or discipline of self-perfection and the first of them is right shakti, the right condition of the powers of the intelligence, heart, vital mind and body. It will only be possible at present to suggest a preliminary perfection of the last of these four, for the full siddhi will have to be dealt with after I have spoken of the supermind and its influence on the rest of the being. The body is not only the necessary outer instrument of the physical part of action, but for the purposes of this life a base or pedestal also for all inner action. All working of mind or spirit has its vibration in the physical consciousness, records itself there in a kind of subordinate corporeal notation and communicates itself to the material world partly at least through the physical machine. But the body of man has natural limitations in this capacity which it imposes on the play of the higher parts of his being. And, secondly, it has a subconscient consciousness of its own in which it keeps with an obstinate fidelity the past habits and past nature of the mental and vital being and which automatically opposes and obstructs any very great upward change or at least prevents it from becoming a radical transformation of the whole nature. It is evident that if we are to have a free divine or spiritual and supramental action conducted by the force and fulfilling the character of a diviner energy, some fairly complete transformation must be effected in this outward character of the bodily nature. The physical being of man has always been felt by the seekers of perfection to be a great impediment and it has been the habit to turn from it with contempt, denial or aversion and a desire to suppress altogether or as far as may be the body and the physical life. But this cannot be the right method for the integral Yoga. The body is given us as one instrument necessary to the totality of our works and it is to be used, not neglected, hurt, suppressed or abolished. If it is imperfect, recalcitrant, obstinate, so are also the other members, the vital being, heart and mind and reason. It has like them to be changed and perfected and to undergo a transformation. As we must get ourselves a new life, new heart, new mind, so we have in a certain sense to build for ourselves a new body.

The first thing the will has to do with the body is to impose on it progressively a new habit of all its being, consciousness, force and outward and inward action. It must be taught an entire passivity in the hands first of the higher instruments, but eventually in the hands of the spirit and its controlling and informing Shakti. It must be accustomed not to impose its own limits on the nobler members, but to shape its action and its response to their demands, to develop, one might say, a higher notation, a higher scale of responses. At present the notation of the body and the physical consciousness has a very large determining power on the music made by this human harp of God; the notes we get from the spirit, from the psychic soul, from the greater life behind our physical life cannot come in freely, cannot develop their high, powerful and proper strain. This condition must be reversed; the body and the physical consciousness must develop the habit of admitting and shaping themselves to these higher strains and not they, but the nobler parts of the nature must determine the music of our life and being.

The control of the body and life by the mind and its thought and will is the first step towards this change. All Yoga implies the carrying of that control to a very high pitch. But afterwards the mind must itself give place to the spirit, to the spiritual force, the supermind and the supramental force. And finally the body must develop a perfect power to hold whatever force is brought into it by the spirit and to contain its action without spilling and wasting it or itself getting cracked. It must be capable of being filled and powerfully used by whatever intensity of spiritual or higher mind or life force without any part of the mechanical instrument being agitated, upset, broken or damaged by the inrush or pressure,—as the brain, vital health or moral nature are often injured in those who unwisely attempt Yogic practice without preparation or by undue means or rashly invite a power they are intellectually, vitally, morally unfit to bear,—and, thus filled, it must have the capacity to work normally, automatically, rightly according to the will of that spiritual or other now unusual agent without distorting, diminishing or mistranslating its intention and stress. This faculty of holding, *dhāraṇa-śakti*, in the physical consciousness, energy and machinery is the most important siddhi or perfection of the body.

The result of these changes will be to make the body a perfect instrument of the spirit. The spiritual force will be able to do what it wills and as it wills in and through the body. It will be able to conduct an unlimited action of the mind or at a higher stage of the supermind without the body betraying the action by fatigue, incapacity, inaptitude or falsification. It will be able too to pour a full tide of the life-force into the body and conduct a large action and joy of the perfected vital being without that quarrel and disparity which is the relation of the normal life-instincts and life-impulses to the insufficient physical instrument they are obliged to use. And it will also be able to conduct a full action of the spiritualised psychic being not falsified, degraded or in any way marred by the lower instincts of the body and to use physical action and expression as a free notation of the higher psychical life. And in the body itself there will be a presence of a greatness of sustaining force, an abounding strength, energy and puissance of outgoing and managing force, a lightness, swiftness and adaptability of the nervous and physical being, a holding and responsive power in the whole physical machine and its driving springs[1] of which it is now even at its strongest and best incapable.

This energy will not be in its essence an outward, physical or muscular strength, but will be of the nature, first, of an unbounded life-power or pranic force, secondly, sustaining and using this pranic energy, a superior or supreme will-power acting in the body. The play of the pranic shakti in the body or form is the condition of all action, even of the most apparently inanimate physical action. It is the universal Prana, as the ancients knew, which in various forms sustains or drives material energy in all physical things from the electron and atom and gas up through the metal, plant, animal, physical man. To get this pranic shakti to act more freely and forcibly in the body is knowingly or unknowingly the attempt of all who strive for a greater perfection of or in the body. The ordinary man tries to command it mechanically by physical exercises and other corporeal means, the Hatha-yogin more greatly and flexibly, but still mechanically by Asana and Pranayama; but for our purpose it can be commanded by more subtle, essential and pliable means; first, by a will in the mind widely opening itself to and potently calling in the universal pranic shakti on which we draw and fixing its stronger presence and more powerful working in the body; secondly, by the will in the mind opening itself rather to the spirit and its power and calling in a higher pranic energy from above, a supramental pranic force; thirdly, the last step, by the highest supramental will of the spirit entering and taking up directly the task of the perfection of the body. In fact, it is always really a will within which drives and makes effective the pranic instrument even when it uses what seem to be purely physical means; but at first it is dependent on the inferior action. When we go higher, the relation is gradually reversed; it is then able to act in its own power or handle the rest only as a subordinate instrumentation.

Most men are not conscious of this pranic force in the body or cannot distinguish it from the more physical form of energy which it informs and uses for its vehicle. But as the consciousness becomes more subtle by practice of Yoga, we can come to be aware of the sea of pranic shakti around us, feel it with the mental consciousness, concretely with a mental sense, see its courses and movements, and direct and act upon it immediately by the will. But until we thus become aware of it, we have to possess a working or at least an experimental faith in its presence and in the power of the will to develop a greater command and use of this prana force. There is necessary a faith, *śraddhā*, in the power of the mind to lay its will on the state and action of the body, such as those have who heal disease by faith, will or mental action; but we must seek this control not only for this or any other limited use, but generally as a legitimate power of the inner and greater over the outer and lesser instrument. This faith is combated by our past habits of mind, by our actual normal experience of its comparative helplessness in our present imperfect system and by an opposing belief in the body and physical consciousness. For they too have a limiting *śraddhā* of their own which opposes the idea in the mind when it seeks to impose on the system the law of a higher yet unattained perfection. But as we persist and find this power giving evidence of itself to our experience, the faith in the mind will be able to found itself more firmly and grow in vigour and the opposing faith in the body will change, admit what it first denied and not only accept in its habits the new yoke but itself call for this higher action. Finally we shall realise the truth that this being we are is or can become whatever it has the faith and will to be,—for faith is only a will aiming at greater truth,— and cease to set limits to our possibility or deny the potential omnipotence of the Self in us, the divine Power working through the human instrument. That however, at least as a practical force, comes in at a later stage of high perfection.

The Prana is not only a force for the action of physical and vital energy, but supports also the mental and spiritual action. Therefore the full and free working of the pranic shakti is required not only for the lower but still necessary use, but also for the free and full operation of mind and supermind and spirit in the instrumentality of our complex human nature. That is the main sense of the use of exercises of Pranayama for control of the vital force and its motions which is so important and indispensable a part of certain systems of Yoga. The same mastery must be got by the seeker of the integral Yoga; but he may arrive at it by other means and in any case he must not be dependent on any physical or breathing exercise for its possession and maintenance, for that will at once bring in a limitation and subjection to Prakriti. Her instrumentation has to be used flexibly by the Purusha, but not to be a fixed control on the Purusha. The necessity of the pranic force, however, remains and will be evident to our self-study and experience. It is in the Vedic image the steed and conveyance of the embodied mind and will, *vāhana*. If it is full of strength and swiftness and a plenitude of all its powers, then the mind can go on the courses of its action with a plenary and unhampered movement. But if it is lame or soon tired or sluggish or weak, then an incapacity is laid on the effectuation of the will and activity of the mind. The same rule holds good of the supermind when it first comes into action. There are indeed states and activities in which the mind takes up the pranic shakti into itself and this dependence is not felt at all; but even then the force is there, though involved in the pure mental energy. The supermind, when it gets into full strength, can do pretty well what it likes with the pranic shakti, and we find that in the end this life power is transformed into the type of a supramentalised prana which is simply one motor power of that greater consciousness. But this belongs to a later stage of the siddhi of the Yoga.

Then again there is the psychic prana, pranic mind or desire soul; this too calls for its own perfection. Here too the first necessity is a fullness of the vital capacity in the mind, its power to do its full work, to take possession of all the impulsions and energies given to our inner psychic life for fulfilment in this existence, to hold them and to be a means for carrying them out with strength, freedom, perfection. Many of the things we need for our perfection, courage, will-power effective in life, all the elements of what we now call force of character and force of personality, depend very largely for their completest strength and spring of energetic action on the fullness of the psychic prana. But along with this fullness there must be an established gladness, clearness and purity in the psychic life-being. This dynamis must not be a troubled, perfervid, stormy, fitfully or crudely passionate strength; energy there must be, rapture of its action it must have, but a clear and glad and pure energy, a seated and firmly supported pure rapture. And as a third condition of its perfection it must be poised in a complete equality. The desire-soul must get rid of the clamour, insistence or inequality of its desires in order that its desires may be satisfied with justice and balance and in the right way and eventually must rid them of the character of desire altogether and change them into impulsion of the divine Ananda. To that end it must make no demands nor seek to impose itself on heart, mind or spirit, but accept with a strong passive and active equality whatever impulsion and command come into it from the spirit through the channel of a still mind and a pure heart. And it must accept too whatever result of the impulse, whatever enjoyment more or less, full or nil, is given to it by the Master of our being. At the same time, possession and enjoyment are its law, function, use, swadharma. It is not intended to be a slain or mortified thing, dull in its receptive power, dreary, suppressed, maimed, inert or null. It must have a full power of possession, a glad power of enjoyment, an exultant power of pure and divine passion and rapture. The enjoyment it will have will be in the essence a spiritual bliss, but one which takes up into itself and transforms the mental, emotional, dynamic, vital and physical joy; it must have therefore an integral capacity for these things and must not by incapacity or fatigue or inability to bear great intensities fail the spirit, mind, heart, will and body. Fullness, clear purity and gladness, equality, capacity for possession and enjoyment are the fourfold perfection of the psychic prana.[2]

The next instrument which needs perfection is the *citta*, and within the complete meaning of this expression we may include the emotional and the pure psychical being. This heart and psychic being of man shot through with the threads of the life instincts is a thing of mixed inconstant colours of emotion and soul vibrations, bad and good, happy and unhappy, satisfied and unsatisfied, troubled and calm, intense and dull. Thus agitated and invaded it is unacquainted with any real peace, incapable of a steady perfection of all its powers. By purification, by equality, by the light of knowledge, by a harmonising of the will it can be brought to a tranquil intensity and perfection. The first two elements of this perfection are on one side a high and large sweetness, openness, gentleness, calm, clarity, on the other side a strong and ardent force and intensity. In the divine no less than in ordinary human character and action there are always two strands, sweetness and strength, mildness and force, *saumya* and *raudra*, the force that bears and harmonises, the force that imposes itself and compels, Vishnu and Ishana, Shiva and Rudra. The two are equally necessary to a perfect world-action. The perversions of the Rudra power in the heart are stormy passion, wrath and fierceness and harshness, hardness, brutality, cruelty, egoistic ambition and love of violence and domination. These and other human perversions have to be got rid of by the flowering of a calm, clear and sweet psychical being.

But on the other hand incapacity of force is also an imperfection. Laxity and weakness, self-indulgence, a certain flabbiness and limpness or inert passivity of the psychical being are the last result of an emotional and psychic life in which energy and power of assertion have been quelled, discouraged or killed. Nor is it a total perfection to have only the strength that endures or to cultivate only a heart of love, charity, tolerance, mildness, meekness and forbearance. The other side of perfection is a self-contained and calm and unegoistic Rudra-power armed with psychic force, the energy of the strong heart which is capable of supporting without shrinking an insistent, an outwardly austere or even, where need is, a violent action. An unlimited light of energy, force, puissance harmonised with sweetness of heart and clarity, capable of being one with it in action, the lightning of Indra starting from the orb of the nectarous moon-rays of Soma is the double perfection. And these two things *saumyatva, tejas*, must base their presence and action on a firm equality of the temperament and of the psychical soul delivered from all crudity and all excess or defect of the heart's light or the heart's power.

Another necessary element is a faith in the heart, a belief in and will to the universal good, an openness to the universal Ananda. The pure psychic being is of the essence of Ananda, it comes from the delight-soul in the universe; but the superficial heart of emotion is overborne by the conflicting appearances of the world and suffers many reactions of grief, fear, depression, passion, short-lived and partial joy. An equal heart is needed for perfection, but not only a passive equality; there must be the sense of a divine power making for good behind all experiences, a faith and will which can turn the poisons of the world to nectar, see the happier spiritual intention behind adversity, the mystery of love behind suffering, the flower of divine strength and joy in the seed of pain. This faith, *kalyāṇa-śraddhā*, is needed in order that the heart and the whole overt psychic being may respond to the secret divine Ananda and change itself into this true original essence. This faith and will must be accompanied by and open into an illimitable widest and intensest capacity for love. For the main business of the heart, its true function is love. It is our destined instrument of complete union and oneness; for to see oneness in the world by the understanding is not enough unless we also feel it with the heart and in the psychic being, and this means a delight in the One and in all existences in the world in him, a love of God and all beings. The heart's faith and will in good are founded on a perception of the one Divine immanent in all things and leading the world. The universal love has to be founded on the heart's sight and psychical and emotional sense of the one Divine, the one Self in all existence. All four elements will then form a unity and even the Rudra power to do battle for the right and the good proceed on the basis of a power of universal love. This is the highest and the most characteristic perfection of the heart, *prema-sāmarthya*.

The last perfection is that of the intelligence and thinking mind, *buddhi*. The first need is the clarity and the purity of the intelligence. It must be freed from the claims of the vital being which seeks to impose the desire of the mind in place of the truth, from the claims of the troubled emotional being which strives to colour, distort, limit and falsify the truth with the hue and shape of the emotions. It must be free too from its own defect, inertia of the thought-power, obstructive narrowness and unwillingness to open to knowledge, intellectual unscrupulousness in thinking, prepossession and preference, self-will in the reason and false determination of the will to knowledge. Its sole will must be to make itself an unsullied mirror of the truth, its essence and its forms and measures and relations, a clear mirror, a just measure, a fine and subtle instrument of harmony, an integral intelligence. This clear and pure intelligence can then become a serene thing of light, a pure and strong radiance emanating from the sun of Truth. But, again, it must become not merely a thing of concentrated dry or white light, but capable of all variety of understanding, supple, rich, flexible, brilliant with all the flame and various with all the colours of the manifestation of the Truth, open to all its forms. And so equipped it will get rid of limitations, not be shut up in this or that faculty or form or working of knowledge, but an instrument ready and capable for whatever work is demanded from it by the Purusha. Purity, clear radiance, rich and flexible variety, integral capacity are the fourfold perfection of the thinking intelligence, *viśuddhi, prakāśa, vicitra-bodha, sarva-jñāna-sāmarthya*.

The normal instruments thus perfected will act each in its own kind without undue interference from each other and serve the unobstructed will of the Purusha in a harmonised totality of our natural being. This perfection must rise constantly in its capacity for action, the energy and force of its working and a certain greatness of the scope of the total nature. They will then be ready for the transformation into their own supramental action in which they will find a more absolute, unified and luminous spiritual truth of the whole perfected nature. The means of this perfection of the instruments we shall have to consider later on; but at present it will be enough to say that the principal conditions are will, self-watching and self-knowledge and a constant practice, *abhyāsa*, of self-modification and transformation. The Purusha has that capacity; for the spirit within can always change and perfect the working of its nature. But the mental being must open the way by a clear and a watchful introspection, an opening of itself to a searching and subtle self-knowledge which will give it the understanding and to an increasing extent the mastery of its natural instruments, a vigilant and insistent will of self-modification and self-transformation—for to that will the Prakriti must with whatever difficulty and whatever initial or prolonged resistance eventually respond,—and an unfailing practice which will constantly reject all defect and perversion and replace it by right state and a right and enhanced working. Askesis, tapasya, patience and faithfulness and rectitude of knowledge and will are the things required until a greater Power than our mental selves directly intervenes to effect a more easy and rapid transformation.

---

1. *mahattva, bala, laghutā, dhāraṇa-sāmarthya.*
2. *pūrṇatā, prasannatā, samatā, bhoga-sāmarthya.*

# SOUL-FORCE AND THE FOURFOLD PERSONALITY

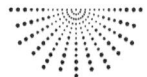

THE PERFECTING of the normal mind, heart, prana and body gives us only the perfection of the psycho-physical machine we have to use and creates certain right instrumental conditions for a divine life and works lived and done with a purer, greater, clearer power and knowledge. The next question is that of the Force which is poured into the instruments, *karaṇa*, and the One who works it for his universal ends. The force at work in us must be the manifest divine Shakti, the supreme or the universal Force unveiled in the liberated individual being, *parā prakṛtir jīvabhūtā*, who will be the doer of all the action and the power of this divine life, *kartā*. The One behind this force will be the Ishwara, the Master of all being, with whom all our existence will be in our perfection a Yoga at once of oneness in being and of union in various relations of the soul and its nature with the Godhead who is seated within us and in whom too we live, move and have our being. It is this Shakti with the Ishwara in her or behind her whose divine presence and way we have to call into all our being and life. For without this divine presence and this greater working there can be no siddhi of the power of the nature.

All the action of man in life is a nexus of the presence of the soul and the workings of Nature, Purusha and Prakriti. The presence and influence of the Purusha represents itself in nature as a certain power of our being which we may call for our immediate purpose soul-force; and it is always this soul-force which supports all the workings of the powers of the reason, the mind, life and body and determines the cast of our conscious being and the type of our nature. The normal ordinarily developed man possesses it in a subdued, a modified, a mechanised, submerged form as temperament and character; but that is only its most outward mould in which Purusha, the conscious soul or being, seems to be limited, conditioned and given some shape by the mechanical Prakriti. The soul flows into whatever moulds of intellectual, ethical, aesthetic, dynamic, vital and physical mind and type the developing nature takes and can act only in the way this formed Prakriti lays on it and move in its narrow groove or relatively wider circle. The man is then sattwic, rajasic or tamasic or a mixture of these qualities and his temperament is only a sort of subtler soul-colour which has been given to the major prominent operation of these fixed modes of his nature. Men of a stronger force get more of the soul-power to the surface and develop what we call a strong or great personality, they have in them something of the Vibhuti as described by the Gita, *vibhūtimat sattvaṁ śrīmad ūrjitam eva vā*, a higher power of being often touched with or sometimes full of some divine afflatus or more than ordinary manifestation of the Godhead which is indeed present in all, even in the weakest or most clouded living being, but here some special force of it begins to come out from behind the veil of the average humanity, and there is something beautiful, attractive, splendid or powerful in these exceptional persons which shines out in their personality, character, life and work. These men too work in the type of their nature-force according to its gunas, but there is something evident in them and yet not easily analysable which is in reality a direct power of the Self and spirit using to strong purpose the mould and direction of the nature. The nature itself thereby rises to or towards a higher grade of its being. Much in the working of the Force may seem egoistic or even perverse, but it is still the touch of the Godhead behind, whatever Daivic, Asuric or even Rakshasic form it may take, which drives the Prakriti and uses it for its own greater purpose. A still more developed power of the being will bring out the real character of this spiritual presence and it will then be seen as something impersonal and self-existent and self-empowered, a sheer soul-force which is other than the mind-force, life-force, force of intelligence, but drives them and, even while following to a certain extent their mould of working, guna, type of nature, yet puts its stamp of an initial transcendence, impersonality, pure fire of spirit, a something beyond the gunas of our normal nature. When the spirit in us is free, then what was behind this soul-force comes out in all its light, beauty and greatness, the Spirit, the Godhead who makes the nature and soul of man his foundation and living representative in cosmic being and mind, action and life.

The Godhead, the spirit manifested in Nature appears in a sea of infinite quality, Ananta-guna. But the executive or mechanical Prakriti is of the threefold guna, sattwa, rajas, tamas, and the Ananta-guna, the spiritual play of infinite quality, modifies itself in this mechanical nature into the type of these three gunas. And in the soul-force in man this Godhead in Nature represents itself as a fourfold effective Power, *catur-vyūha*, a Power for knowledge, a Power for strength, a Power for mutuality and active and productive relation and interchange, a Power for works and labour and service, and its presence casts all human life into a nexus and inner and outer operation of these four things. The ancient thought of India conscious of this fourfold type of active human personality and nature built out of it the four types of the Brahmana, Kshatriya, Vaishya and Shudra, each with its spiritual turn, ethical ideal, suitable upbringing, fixed function in society and place in the evolutionary scale of the spirit. As always tends to be the case when we too much externalise and mechanise the more subtle truths of our nature, this became a hard and fast system inconsistent with the freedom and variability and complexity of the finer developing spirit in man. Nevertheless the truth behind it exists and is one of some considerable importance in the perfection of our power of nature; but we have to take it in its inner aspects, first, personality, character, temperament, soul-type, then the soul-force which lies behind them and wears these forms, and lastly the play of the free spiritual Shakti in which they find their culmination and unity beyond all modes. For the crude external idea that a man is born as a Brahmana, Kshatriya, Vaishya or Shudra and that alone, is not a psychological truth of our being. The psychological fact is that there are these four active powers and tendencies of the Spirit and its executive Shakti within us and the predominance of one or the other in the more well-formed part of our personality gives us our main tendencies, dominant qualities and capacities, effective turn in action and life. But they are more or less present in all men, here manifest, there latent, here developed, there subdued and depressed or subordinate, and in the perfect man will be raised up to a fullness and harmony which in the spiritual freedom will burst out into the free play of the infinite quality of the spirit in the inner and outer life and in the self-enjoying creative play of the Purusha with his and the world's Nature-Power.

The most outward psychological form of these things is the mould or trend of the nature towards certain dominant tendencies, capacities, characteristics, form of active power, quality of the mind and inner life, cultural personality or type. The turn is often towards the predominance of the intellectual element and the capacities which make for the seeking and finding of knowledge and an intellectual creation or formativeness and a preoccupation with ideas and the study of ideas or of life and the information and development of the reflective intelligence. According to the grade of the development there is produced successively the make and character of the man of active, open, inquiring intelligence, then the intellectual and, last, the thinker, sage, great mind of knowledge. The soul-powers which make their appearance by a considerable development of this temperament, personality, soul-type, are a mind of light more and more open to all ideas and knowledge and incomings of Truth; a hunger and passion for knowledge, for its growth in ourselves, for its communication to others, for its reign in the world, the reign of reason and right and truth and justice and, on a higher level of the harmony of our greater being, the reign of the spirit and its universal unity and light and love; a power of this light in the mind and will which makes all the life subject to reason and its right and truth or to the spirit and spiritual right and truth and subdues the lower members to their greater law; a poise in the temperament turned from the first to patience, steady musing and calm, to reflection, to meditation, which dominates and quiets the turmoil of the will and passions and makes for high thinking and pure living, founds the self-governed sattwic mind, grows into a more and more mild, lofty, impersonalised and universalised personality. This is the ideal character and soul-power of the Brahmana, the priest of knowledge. If it is not there in all its sides, we have the imperfections or perversions of the type, a mere intellectuality or curiosity for ideas without ethical or other elevation, a narrow concentration on some kind of intellectual activity without the greater needed openness of mind, soul and spirit, or the arrogance and exclusiveness of the intellectual shut up in his intellectuality, or an ineffective idealism without any hold on life, or any other of the characteristic incompletenesses and limitations of the intellectual, religious, scientific or philosophic mind. These are stoppings short on the way or temporary exclusive concentrations, but a fullness of the divine soul and power of truth and knowledge in man is the perfection of this Dharma or Swabhava, the accomplished Brahminhood of the complete Brahmana.

On the other hand the turn of the nature may be to the predominance of the will-force and the capacities which make for strength, energy, courage, leadership, protection, rule, victory in every kind of battle, a creative and formative action, the will-power which lays its hold on the material of life and on the wills of other men and compels the environment into the shapes which the Shakti within us seeks to impose on life or acts powerfully according to the work to be done to maintain what is in being or to destroy it and make clear the paths of the world or to bring out into definite shape what is to be. This may be there in lesser or greater power or form and according to its grade and force we have successively the mere fighter or man of action, the man of self-imposing active will and personality and the ruler, conqueror, leader of a cause, creator, founder in whatever field of the active formation of life. The various imperfections of the soul and mind produce many imperfections and perversities of this type,—the man of mere brute force of will, the worshipper of power without any other ideal or higher purpose, the selfish, dominant personality, the aggressive violent rajasic man, the grandiose egoist, the Titan, Asura, Rakshasa. But the soul-powers to which this type of nature opens on its higher grades are as necessary as those of the Brahmana to the perfection of our human nature. The high fearlessness which no danger or difficulty can daunt and which feels its power equal to meet and face and bear whatever assault of man or fortune or adverse gods, the dynamic audacity and daring which shrinks from no adventure or enterprise as beyond the powers of a human soul free from disabling weakness and fear, the love of honour which would scale the heights of the highest nobility of man and stoop to nothing little, base, vulgar or weak, but maintains untainted the ideal of high courage, chivalry, truth, straightforwardness, sacrifice of the lower to the higher self, helpfulness to men, unflinching resistance to injustice and oppression, self-control and mastery, noble leading, warriorhood and captainship of the journey and the battle, the high self-confidence of power, capacity, character and courage indispensable to the man of action,—these are the things that build the make of the Kshatriya. To carry these things to their highest degree and give them a certain divine fullness, purity and grandeur is the perfection of those who have this Swabhava and follow this Dharma.

A third turn is one that brings out into relief the practical arranging intelligence and the instinct of life to produce, exchange, possess, enjoy, contrive, put things in order and balance, spend itself and get and give and take, work out to the best advantage the active relations of existence. In its outward action it is this power that appears as the skilful devising intelligence, the legal, professional, commercial, industrial, economical, practical and scientific, mechanical, technical and utilitarian mind. This nature is accompanied at the normal level of its fullness by a general temperament which is at once grasping and generous, prone to amass and treasure, to enjoy, show and use, bent upon efficient exploitation of the world or its surroundings, but well capable too of practical philanthropy, humanity, ordered benevolence, orderly and ethical by rule but without any high distinction of the finer ethical spirit, a mind of the middle levels, not straining towards the heights, not great to break and create noble moulds of life, but marked by capacity, adaptation and measure. The powers, limitations and perversions of this type are familiar to us on a large scale, because this is the very spirit which has made our modern commercial and industrial civilisation. But if we look at the greater inner capacities and soul-values, we shall find that here also there are things that enter into the completeness of human perfection. The Power that thus outwardly expresses itself on our present lower levels is one that can throw itself out in the great utilities of life and at its freest and widest makes, not for oneness and identity which is the highest reach of knowledge or the mastery and spiritual kingship which is the highest reach of strength, but still for something which is also essential to the wholeness of existence, equal mutuality and the exchange of soul with soul and life with life. Its powers are, first, a skill, *kauśala*, which fashions and obeys law, recognises the uses and limits of relations, adapts itself to settled and developing movements, produces and perfects the outer technique of creation and action and life, assures possession and proceeds from possession to growth, is watchful over order and careful in progress and makes the most of the material of existence and its means and ends; then a power of self-spending skilful in lavishness and skilful in economy, which recognises the great law of interchange and amasses in order to throw out in a large return, increasing the currents of interchange and the fruitfulness of existence; a power of giving and ample creative liberality, mutual helpfulness and utility to others which becomes the source in an open soul of just beneficence, humanitarianism, altruism of a practical kind; finally, a power of enjoyment, a productive, possessive, active opulence luxurious of the prolific Ananda of existence. A largeness of mutuality, a generous fullness of the relations of life, a lavish self-spending and return and ample interchange between existence and existence, a full enjoyment and use of the rhythm and balance of fruitful and productive life are the perfection of those who have this Swabhava and follow this Dharma.

The other turn is towards work and service. This was in the old order the dharma or soul-type of the Shudra and the Shudra in that order was considered as not one of the twice-born, but an inferior type. A more recent consideration of the values of existence lays stress on the dignity of labour and sees in its toil the bed-rock of the relations between man and man. There is a truth in both attitudes. For this force in the material world is at once in its necessity the foundation of material existence or rather that on which it moves, the feet of the creator Brahma in the old parable, and in its primal state not uplifted by knowledge, mutuality or strength a thing which reposes on instinct, desire and inertia. The well-developed Shudra soul-type has the instinct of toil and the capacity of labour and service; but toil as opposed to easy or natural action is a thing imposed on the natural man which he bears because without it he cannot assure his existence or get his desires and he has to force himself or be forced by others or circumstances to spend himself in work. The natural Shudra works not from a sense of the dignity of labour or from the enthusiasm of service,—though that comes by the cultivation of his dharma,—not as the man of knowledge for the joy or gain of knowledge, not from a sense of honour, nor as the born craftsman or artist for love of his work or ardour for the beauty of its technique, nor from an ordered sense of mutuality or large utility, but for the maintenance of his existence and gratification of his primal wants, and when these are satisfied, he indulges, if left to himself, his natural indolence, the indolence which is normal to the tamasic quality in all of us, but comes out most clearly in the uncompelled primitive man, the savage. The unregenerated Shudra is born therefore for service rather than for free labour and his temperament is prone to an inert ignorance, a gross unthinking self-indulgence of the instincts, a servility, an unreflective obedience and mechanical discharge of duty varied by indolence, evasion, spasmodic revolt, an instinctive and uninformed life. The ancients held that all men are born in their lower nature as Shudras and only regenerated by ethical and spiritual culture, but in their highest inner self are Brahmanas capable of the full spirit and godhead, a theory which is not far perhaps from the psychological truth of our nature.

And yet when the soul develops, it is in this Swabhava and Dharma of work and service that there are found some of the most necessary and beautiful elements of our greatest perfection and the key to much of the secret of the highest spiritual evolution. For the soul powers that belong to the full development of this force in us are of the greatest importance, —the power of service to others, the will to make our life a thing of work and use to God and man, to obey and follow and accept whatever great influence and needful discipline, the love which consecrates service, a love which asks for no return, but spends itself for the satisfaction of that which we love, the power to bring down this love and service into the physical field and the desire to give our body and life as well as our soul and mind and will and capacity to God and man, and, as a result, the power of complete self-surrender, *ātma-samarpaṇa*, which transferred to the spiritual life becomes one of the greatest most revealing keys to freedom and perfection. In these things lies the perfection of this Dharma and the nobility of this Swabhava. Man could not be perfect and complete if he had not this element of nature in him to raise to its divine power.

None of these four types of personality can be complete even in its own field if it does not bring into it something of the other qualities. The man of knowledge cannot serve Truth with freedom and perfection, if he has not intellectual and moral courage, will, audacity, the strength to open and conquer new kingdoms, otherwise he becomes a slave of the limited intellect or a servant or at most a ritual priest of only an established knowledge,[1]—cannot use his knowledge to the best advantage unless he has the adaptive skill to work out its truths for the practice of life, otherwise he lives only in the idea,—cannot make the entire consecration of his knowledge unless he has the spirit of service to humanity, to the Godhead in man and the Master of his being. The man of power must illumine and uplift and govern his force and strength by knowledge, light of reason or religion or the spirit, otherwise he becomes the mere forceful Asura,—must have the skill which will help him best to use and administer and regulate his strength and make it creative and fruitful and adapted to his relations with others, otherwise it becomes a mere drive of force across the field of life, a storm that passes and devastates more than it constructs,—must be capable too of obedience and make the use of his strength a service to God and the world, otherwise he becomes a selfish dominator, tyrant, brutal compeller of men's souls and bodies. The man of productive mind and work must have an open inquiring mind and ideas and knowledge, otherwise he moves in the routine of his functions without expansive growth, must have courage and enterprise, must bring a spirit of service into his getting and production, in order that he may not only get but give, not only amass and enjoy his own life, but consciously help the fruitfulness and fullness of the surrounding life by which he profits. The man of labour and service becomes a helpless drudge and slave of society if he does not bring knowledge and honour and aspiration and skill into his work, since only so can he rise by an opening mind and will and understanding usefulness to the higher dharmas. But the greater perfection of man comes when he enlarges himself to include all these powers, even though one of them may lead the others, and opens his nature more and more into the rounded fullness and universal capacity of the fourfold spirit. Man is not cut out into an exclusive type of one of these dharmas, but all these powers are in him at work at first in an ill-formed confusion, but he gives shape to one or another in birth after birth, progresses from one to the other even in the same life and goes on towards the total development of his inner existence. Our life itself is at once an inquiry after truth and knowledge, a struggle and battle of our will with ourselves and surrounding forces, a constant production, adaptation, application of skill to the material of life and a sacrifice and service.

These things are the ordinary aspects of the soul while it is working out its force in nature, but when we get nearer to our inner selves, then we get too a glimpse and experience of something which was involved in these forms and can disengage itself and stand behind and drive them, as if a general Presence or Power brought to bear on the particular working of this living and thinking machine. This is the force of the soul itself presiding over and filling the powers of its nature. The difference is that the first way is personal in its stamp, limited and determined in its action and mould, dependent on the instrumentation, but here there emerges something impersonal in the personal form, independent and self-sufficient even in the use of the instrumentation, indeterminable though determining both itself and things, something which acts with a much greater power upon the world and uses particular power only as one means of communication and impact on man and circumstance. The Yoga of self-perfection brings out this soul-force and gives it its largest scope, takes up all the fourfold powers and throws them into the free circle of an integral and harmonious spiritual dynamis. The godhead, the soul-power of knowledge rises to the highest degree of which the individual nature can be the supporting basis. A free mind of light develops which is open to every kind of revelation, inspiration, intuition, idea, discrimination, thinking synthesis; an enlightened life of the mind grasps at all knowledge with a delight of finding and reception and holding, a spiritual enthusiasm, passion, or ecstasy; a power of light full of spiritual force, illumination and purity of working manifests its empire, *brahmatejas*, *brahma-varcas*; a bottomless steadiness and illimitable calm upholds all the illumination, movement, action as on some rock of ages, equal, unperturbed, unmoved, *acyuta*.

The godhead, the soul-power of will and strength rises to a like largeness and altitude. An absolute calm fearlessness of the free spirit, an infinite dynamic courage which no peril, limitation of possibility, wall of opposing force can deter from pursuing the work or aspiration imposed by the spirit, a high nobility of soul and will untouched by any littleness or baseness and moving with a certain greatness of step to spiritual victory or the success of the God-given work through whatever temporary defeat or obstacle, a spirit never depressed or cast down from faith and confidence in the power that works in the being, are the signs of this perfection. There comes too to fulfilment a large godhead, a soul-power of mutuality, a free self-spending and spending of gift and possession in the work to be done, lavished for the production, the creation, the achievement, the possession, gain, utilisable return, a skill that observes the law and adapts the relation and keeps the measure, a great taking into oneself from all beings and a free giving out of oneself to all, a divine commerce, a large enjoyment of the mutual delight of life. And finally there comes to perfection the godhead, the soul-power of service, the universal love that lavishes itself without demand of return, the embrace that takes to itself the body of God in man and works for help and service, the abnegation that is ready to bear the yoke of the Master and make the life a free servitude to Him and under his direction to the claim and need of his creatures, the self-surrender of the whole being to the Master of our being and his work in the world. These things unite, assist and enter into each other, become one. The full consummation comes in the greatest souls most capable of perfection, but some large manifestation of this fourfold soul-power must be sought and can be attained by all who practise the integral Yoga.

These are the signs, but behind is the soul which thus expresses itself in a consummation of nature. And this soul is an out-coming of the free self of the liberated man. That self is of no character, being infinite, but bears and upholds the play of all character, supports a kind of infinite, one, yet multiple personality, *nirguṇo guṇī*, is in its manifestation capable of infinite quality, *anantaguṇa*. The force that it uses is the supreme and universal, the divine and infinite Shakti pouring herself into the individual being and freely determining action for the divine purpose.

---

1. That perhaps is why it was the Kshatriya bringing his courage, audacity, spirit of conquest into the fields of intuitive knowledge and spiritual experience who first discovered the great truths of Vedanta.

# THE DIVINE SHAKTI

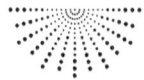

THE RELATION between the Purusha and Prakriti which emerges as one advances in the Yoga of self-perfection is the next thing that we have to understand carefully in this part of the Yoga. In the spiritual truth of our being the power which we call Nature is the power of being, consciousness and will and therefore the power of self-expression and self-creation of the self, soul or Purusha. But to our ordinary mind in the ignorance and to its experience of things the force of Prakriti has a different appearance. When we look at it in its universal action outside ourselves, we see it first as a mechanical energy in the cosmos which acts upon matter or in its own created forms of matter. In matter it evolves powers and processes of life and in living matter powers and processes of mind. Throughout its operations it acts by fixed laws and in each kind of created thing displays varying properties of energy and laws of process which give its character to the genus or species and again in the individual develops without infringing the law of the kind minor characteristics and variations of a considerable consequence. It is this mechanical appearance of Prakriti which has preoccupied the modern scientific mind and made for it its whole view of Nature, and so much so that science still hopes and labours with a very small amount of success to explain all phenomena of life by laws of matter and all phenomena of mind by laws of living matter. Here soul or spirit has no place and nature cannot be regarded as power of spirit.

Since the whole of our existence is mechanical, physical and bounded by the biological phenomenon of a brief living consciousness and man is a creature and instrument of material energy, the spiritual self-evolution of Yoga can be only a delusion, hallucination, abnormal state of mind or self-hypnosis. In any case it cannot be what it represents itself to be, a discovery of the eternal truth of our being and a passing above the limited truth of the mental, vital and physical to the full truth of our spiritual nature.

But when we look, not at external mechanical Nature to the exclusion of our personality, but at the inner subjective experience of man the mental being, our nature takes to us a quite different appearance. We may believe intellectually in a purely mechanical view even of our subjective existence, but we cannot act upon it or make it quite real to our self-experience. For we are conscious of an I which does not seem identical with our nature, but capable of a standing back from it, of a detached observation and criticism and creative use of it, and of a will which we naturally think of as a free will; and even if this be a delusion, we are still obliged in practice to act as if we were responsible mental beings capable of a free choice of our actions, able to use or misuse and to turn to higher or lower ends our nature. And even we seem to be struggling both with our environmental and with our own present nature and striving to get mastery over a world which imposes itself on and masters us and at the same time to become something more than we now are. But the difficulty is that we are only in command, if at all, over a small part of ourselves, the rest is subconscient or subliminal and beyond our control, our will acts only in a small selection of our activities; the most is a process of mechanism and habit and we must strive constantly with ourselves and surrounding circumstances to make the least advance or self-amelioration. There seems to be a dual being in us; Soul and Nature, Purusha and Prakriti, seem to be half in agreement, half at odds, Nature laying its mechanical control on the soul, the soul attempting to change and master nature. And the question is what is the fundamental character of this duality and what the issue.

The Sankhya explanation is that our present existence is governed by a dual principle. Prakriti is inert without the contact of Purusha, acts only by a junction with it and then too by the fixed mechanism of her instruments and qualities; Purusha, passive and free apart from Prakriti, becomes by contact with her and sanction to her works subject to this mechanism, lives in her limitation of ego-sense and must get free by withdrawing the sanction and returning to its own proper principle. Another explanation that tallies with a certain part of our experience is that there is a dual being in us, the animal and material, or more widely the lower nature-bound, and the soul or spiritual being entangled by mind in the material existence or in world-nature, and freedom comes by escape from the entanglement, the soul returning to its native planes or the self or spirit to its pure existence. The perfection of the soul then is to be found not at all in, but beyond Nature.

But in a higher than our present mental consciousness we find that this duality is only a phenomenal appearance. The highest and real truth of existence is the one Spirit, the supreme Soul, Purushottama, and it is the power of being of this Spirit which manifests itself in all that we experience as universe. This universal Nature is not a lifeless, inert or unconscious mechanism, but informed in all its movements by the universal Spirit. The mechanism of its process is only an outward appearance and the reality is the Spirit creating or manifesting its own being by its own power of being in all that is in Nature. Soul and Nature in us too are only a dual appearance of the one existence. The universal energy acts in us, but the soul limits itself by the ego-sense, lives in a partial and separate experience of her workings, uses only a modicum and a fixed action of her energy for its self-expression. It seems rather to be mastered and used by this energy than to use it, because it identifies itself with the ego-sense which is part of the natural instrumentation and lives in the ego experience. The ego is in fact driven by the mechanism of Nature of which it is a part and the ego-will is not and cannot be a free will. To arrive at freedom, mastery and perfection we have to get back to the real self and soul within and arrive too thereby at our true relations with our own and with universal nature.

In our active being this translates itself into a replacement of our egoistic, our personal, our separatively individual will and energy by a universal and a divine will and energy which determines our action in harmony with the universal action and reveals itself as the direct will and the all-guiding power of the Purushottama. We replace the inferior action of the limited, ignorant and imperfect personal will and energy in us by the action of the divine Shakti. To open ourselves to the universal energy is always possible to us, because that is all around us and always flowing into us, it is that which supports and supplies all our inner and outer action and in fact we have no power of our own in any separately individual sense, but only a personal formulation of the one Shakti. And on the other hand this universal Shakti is within ourselves, concentrated in us, for the whole power of it is present in each individual as in the universe, and there are means and processes by which we can awaken its greater and potentially infinite force and liberate it to its larger workings.

We can become aware of the existence and presence of the universal Shakti in the various forms of her power. At present we are conscious only of the power as formulated in our physical mind, nervous being and corporeal case sustaining our various activities. But if we can once get beyond this first formation by some liberation of the hidden, recondite, subliminal parts of our existence by Yoga, we become aware of a greater life force, a pranic Shakti, which supports and fills the body and supplies all the physical and vital activities,—for the physical energy is only a modified form of this force,—and supplies and sustains too from below all our mental action. This force we feel in ourselves also, but we can feel it too around us and above, one with the same energy in us, and can draw it in and down to aggrandise our normal action or call upon and get it to pour into us. It is an illimitable ocean of Shakti and will pour as much of itself as we can hold into our being. This pranic force we can use for any of the activities of life, body or mind with a far greater and effective power than any that we command in our present operations, limited as they are by the physical formula. The use of this pranic power liberates us from that limitation to the extent of our ability to use it in place of the body-bound energy. It can be used so to direct the prana as to manage more powerfully or to rectify any bodily state or action, as to heal illness or to get rid of fatigue, and to liberate an enormous amount of mental exertion and play of will or knowledge. The exercises of Pranayama are the familiar mechanical means of freeing and getting control of the pranic energy. They heighten too and set free the psychic, mental and spiritual energies which ordinarily depend for their opportunity of action on the pranic force. But the same thing can be done by mental will and practice or by an increasing opening of ourselves to a higher spiritual power of the Shakti. The pranic Shakti can be directed not only upon ourselves, but effectively towards others or on things or happenings for whatever purposes the will dictates. Its effectivity is immense, in itself illimitable, and limited only by defect of the power, purity and universality of the spiritual or other will which is brought to bear upon it; but still, however great and powerful, it is a lower formulation, a link between the mind and body, an instrumental force. There is a consciousness in it, a presence of the spirit, of which we are aware, but it is encased, involved in and preoccupied with the urge to action. It is not to this action of the Shakti that we can leave the whole burden of our activities; we have either to use its lendings by our own enlightened personal will or else call in a higher guidance; for of itself it will act with greater force, but still according to our imperfect nature and mainly by the drive and direction of the life-power in us and not according to the law of the highest spiritual existence.

The ordinary power by which we govern the pranic energy is that of the embodied mind. But when we get clear above the physical mind, we can get too above the pranic force to the consciousness of a pure mental energy which is a higher formulation of the Shakti. There we are aware of a universal mind consciousness closely associated with this energy in, around and above us,—above, that is to say, the level of our ordinary mind status,—giving all the substance and shaping all the forms of our will and knowledge and of the psychic element in our impulses and emotions. This mind force can be made to act upon the pranic energy and can impose upon it the influence, colour, shape, character, direction of our ideas, our knowledge, our more enlightened volition and thus more effectively bring our life and vital being into harmony with our higher powers of being, ideals and spiritual aspirations. In our ordinary state these two, the mental and the pranic being and energies, are very much mixed up and run into each other, and we are not able clearly to distinguish them or get a full hold of the one on the other and so control effectively the lower by the higher and more understanding principle. But when we take our station above the physical mind, we are able then to separate clearly the two forms of energy, the two levels of our being, disentangle their action and act with a clearer and more potent self-knowledge and an enlightened and a purer will-power. Nevertheless the control is not complete, spontaneous, sovereign so long as we work with the mind as our chief guiding and controlling force. The mental energy we find to be itself derivative, a lower and limiting power of the conscious spirit which acts only by isolated and combined seeings, imperfect and incomplete half-lights which we take for full and adequate light, and with a disparity between the idea and knowledge and the effective will-power. And we are aware soon of a far higher power of the Spirit and its Shakti concealed or above, superconscient to mind or partially acting through the mind, of which all this is an inferior derivation.

The Purusha and Prakriti are on the mental level as in the rest of our being closely joined and much involved in each other and we are not able to distinguish clearly soul and nature. But in the purer substance of mind we can more easily discern the dual strain. The mental Purusha is naturally able in its own native principle of mind to detach itself, as we have seen, from the workings of its Prakriti and there is then a division of our being between a consciousness that observes and can reserve its will-power and an energy full of the substance of consciousness that takes the forms of knowledge, will and feeling. This detachment gives at its highest a certain freedom from the compulsion of the soul by its mental nature. For ordinarily we are driven and carried along in the stream of our own and the universal active energy partly floundering in its waves, partly maintaining and seeming to guide or at least propel ourselves by a collected thought and an effort of the mental will muscle; but now there is a part of ourselves, nearest to the pure essence of self, which is free from the stream, can quietly observe and to a certain extent decide its immediate movement and course and to a greater extent its ultimate direction. The Purusha can at last act upon the Prakriti from half apart, from behind or from above her as a presiding person or presence, *adhyakṣa*, by the power of sanction and control inherent in the spirit.

What we shall do with this relative freedom depends on our aspiration, our idea of the relation we must have with our highest self, with God and Nature. It is possible for the Purusha to use it on the mental plane itself for a constant self-observation, self-development, self-modification, to sanction, reject, alter, bring out new formulations of the nature and establish a calm and disinterested action, a high and pure sattwic balance and rhythm of its energy, a personality perfected in the sattwic principle. This may amount only to a highly mentalised perfection of our present intelligence and the ethical and the psychic being or else, aware of the greater self in us, it may impersonalise, universalise, spiritualise its self-conscious existence and the action of its nature and arrive either at a large quietude or a large perfection of the spiritualised mental energy of its being. It is possible again for the Purusha to stand back entirely and by a refusal of sanction allow the whole normal action of the mind to exhaust itself, run down, spend its remaining impetus of habitual action and fall into silence. Or else this silence may be imposed on the mental energy by rejection of its action and a constant command to quietude. The soul may through the confirmation of this quietude and mental silence pass into some ineffable tranquillity of the spirit and vast cessation of the activities of Nature. But it is also possible to make this silence of the mind and ability to suspend the habits of the lower nature a first step towards the discovery of a superior formulation, a higher grade of the status and energy of our being and pass by an ascent and transformation into the supramental power of the spirit. And this may even, though with more difficulty, be done without resorting to the complete state of quietude of the normal mind by a persistent and progressive transformation of all the mental into their greater corresponding supramental powers and activities. For everything in the mind derives from and is a limited, inferior, groping, partial or perverse translation into mentality of something in the supermind. But neither of these movements can be successfully executed by the sole individual unaided power of the mental Purusha in us, but needs the help, intervention and guidance of the divine Self, the Ishwara, the Purushottama. For the supermind is the divine mind and it is on the supramental plane that the individual arrives at his right, integral, luminous and perfect relation with the supreme and universal Purusha and the supreme and universal Para Prakriti.

As the mind progresses in purity, capacity of stillness or freedom from absorption in its own limited action, it becomes aware of and is able to reflect, bring into itself or enter into the conscious presence of the Self, the supreme and universal Spirit, and it becomes aware too of grades and powers of the spirit higher than its own highest ranges. It becomes aware of an infinite of the consciousness of being, an infinite ocean of all the power and energy of illimitable consciousness, an infinite ocean of Ananda, of the self-moved delight of existence. It may be aware of one or other only of these things, for the mind can separate and feel exclusively as distinct original principles what in a higher experience are inseparable powers of the One, or it may feel them in a trinity or fusion which reveals or arrives at their oneness. It may become aware of it on the side of Purusha or on the side of Prakriti. On the side of Purusha it reveals itself as Self or Spirit, as Being or as the one sole existent Being, the divine Purushottama, and the individual Jiva soul can enter into entire oneness with it in its timeless self or in its universality, or enjoy nearness, immanence, difference without any gulf of separation and enjoy too inseparably and at one and the same time oneness of being and delight-giving difference of relation in active experiencing nature. On the side of Prakriti the power and Ananda of the Spirit come into the front to manifest this Infinite in the beings and personalities and ideas and forms and forces of the universe and there is then present to us the divine

Mahashakti, original Power, supreme Nature, holding in herself infinite existence and creating the wonders of the cosmos. The mind grows conscious of this illimitable ocean of Shakti or else of her presence high above the mind and pouring something of herself into us to constitute all that we are and think and will and do and feel and experience, or it is conscious of her all around us and our personality a wave of the ocean of power of spirit, or of her presence in us and of her action there based on our present form of natural existence but originated from above and raising us towards the higher spiritual status. The mind too can rise towards and touch her infinity or merge itself in it in trance of samadhi or can lose itself in her universality, and then our individuality disappears, our centre of action is then no longer in us, but either outside our bodied selves or nowhere; our mental activities are then no longer our own, but come into this frame of mind, life and body from the universal, work themselves out and pass leaving no impression on us, and this frame of ourselves too is only an insignificant circumstance in her cosmic vastness. But the perfection sought in the integral Yoga is not only to be one with her in her highest spiritual power and one with her in her universal action, but to realise and possess the fullness of this Shakti in our individual being and nature. For the supreme Spirit is one as Purusha or as Prakriti, conscious being or power of conscious being, and as the Jiva in essence of self and spirit is one with the supreme Purusha, so on the side of Nature, in power of self and spirit it is one with Shakti, *parā prakṛtir jīvabhūtā*. To realise this double oneness is the condition of the integral self-perfection. The Jiva is then the meeting-place of the play of oneness of the supreme Soul and Nature.

To reach this perfection we have to become aware of the divine Shakti, draw her to us and call her in to fill the whole system and take up the charge of all our activities. There will then be no separate personal will or individual energy trying to conduct our actions, no sense of a little personal self as the doer, nor will it be the lower energy of the three gunas, the mental, vital and physical nature. The divine Shakti will fill us and preside over and take up all our inner activities, our outer life, our Yoga. She will take up the mental energy, her own lower formation, and raise it to its highest and purest and fullest powers of intelligence and will and psychic action. She will change the mechanical energies of the mind, life and body which now govern us into delight-filled manifestations of her own living and conscious power and presence. She will manifest in us and relate to each other all the various spiritual experiences of which the mind is capable. And as the crown of this process she will bring down the supramental light into the mental levels, change the stuff of mind into the stuff of supermind, transform all the lower energies into energies of her supramental nature and raise us into our being of gnosis. The Shakti will reveal herself as the power of the Purushottama, and it is the Ishwara who will manifest himself in his force of supermind and spirit and be the master of our being, action, life and Yoga.

# THE ACTION OF THE DIVINE SHAKTI

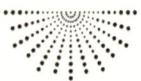

THIS IS the nature of the divine Shakti that it is the timeless power of the Divine which manifests itself in time as a universal force creating, constituting, maintaining and directing all the movements and workings of the universe. This universal Power is apparent to us first on the lower levels of existence as a mental, vital and material cosmic energy of which all our mental, vital and physical activities are the operations. It is necessary for our sadhana that we should thoroughly realise this truth in order to escape from the pressure of the limiting ego view and universalise ourselves even on these lower levels where ordinarily the ego reigns in full force. To see that we are not the originators of action but that it is rather this Power that acts in ourselves and in all others, not I and others the doers, but the one Prakriti, which is the rule of the Karma-yoga, is also the right rule here. The ego sense serves to limit, separate and sharply differentiate, to make the most of the individual form and it is there because it is indispensable to the evolution of the lower life. But when we would rise above to a higher divine life we must loosen the force of the ego and eventually get rid of it —as for the lower life the development of ego, so for the higher life this reverse movement of elimination of the ego is indispensable. To see our actions as not our own but those of the divine Shakti working in the form of the lower Prakriti on the inferior levels of the conscious being, helps powerfully towards this change. And if we can do this, then the separation of our mental, vital and physical consciousness from that of other beings thins and lessens; the limitations of its workings remain indeed, but they are broadened and taken up into a large sense and vision of the universal working; the specialising and individualising differentiations of Nature abide for their own proper purpose, but are no longer a prison. The individual feels his mind, life and physical existence to be one with that of others amid all differences and one with the total power of the spirit in Nature.

This however is a stage and not the whole perfection. The existence, however comparatively large and free, is still subject to the inferior nature. The sattwic, rajasic and tamasic ego is diminished but not eliminated; or if it seems to disappear, it has only sunk in our parts of action into the universal operation of the gunas, remains involved in them and is still working in a covert, subconscient fashion and may force itself to the front at any time. The sadhaka has therefore first to keep the idea and get the realisation of a one self or spirit in all behind all these workings. He must be aware behind Prakriti of the one supreme and universal Purusha. He must see and feel not only that all is the self-shaping of the one Force, Prakriti or Nature, but that all her actions are those of the Divine in all, the one Godhead in all, however veiled, altered and as it were perverted—for perversion comes by a conversion into lower forms —by transmission through the ego and the gunas. This will farther diminish the open or covert insistence of the ego and, if thoroughly realised, it will make it difficult or impossible for it to assert itself in such a way as to disturb or hamper the farther progress. The ego-sense will become, so far as it interferes at all, a foreign intrusive element and only a fringe of the mist of the old ignorance hanging on to the outskirts of the consciousness and its action. And, secondly, the universal Shakti must be realised, must be seen and felt and borne in the potent purity of its higher action, its supramental and spiritual workings. This greater vision of the Shakti will enable us to escape from the control of the gunas, to convert them into their divine equivalents and dwell in a consciousness in which the Purusha and Prakriti are one and not separated or hidden in or behind each other. There the Shakti will be in its every movement evident to us and naturally, spontaneously, irresistibly felt as nothing else but the active presence of the Divine, the shape of power of the supreme Self and Spirit.

The Shakti in this higher status reveals itself as the presence or potentiality of the infinite existence, consciousness, will, delight, and when it is so seen and felt, the being turns towards it in whatever way, with its adoration or its will of aspiration or some kind of attraction of the lesser to the greater, to know it, to be full of and possessed by it, to be one with it in the sense and action of the whole nature. But at first while we still live in the mind, there is a gulf of division or else a double action. The mental, vital and physical energy in us and the universe is felt to be a derivation from the supreme Shakti, but at the same time an inferior, separated and in some sense another working. The real spiritual force may send down its messages or the light and power of its presence above us to the lower levels or may descend occasionally and even for a time possess, but it is then mixed with the inferior workings and partially transforms and spiritualises them, but is itself diminished and altered in the process. There is an intermittent higher action or a dual working of the nature. Or we find that the Shakti for a time raises the being to a higher spiritual plane and then lowers it back into the inferior levels. These alternations must be regarded as the natural vicissitudes of a process of transformation from the normal to the spiritual being. The transformation, the perfection cannot for the integral Yoga be complete until the link between the mental and the spiritual action is formed and a higher knowledge applied to all the activities of our existence. That link is the supramental or gnostic energy in which the incalculable infinite power of the supreme being, consciousness, delight formulates itself as an ordering divine will and wisdom, a light and power in the being which shapes all the thought, will, feeling, action and replaces the corresponding individual movements.

This supramental Shakti may form itself as a spiritualised intuitive light and power in the mind itself, and that is a great but still a mentally limited spiritual action. Or it may transform altogether the mind and raise the whole being to the supramental level. In any case this is the first necessity of this part of the Yoga, to lose the ego of the doer, the ego idea and the sense of one's own power of action and initiation of action and control of the result of action and merge it in the sense and vision of the universal Shakti originating, shaping, turning to its ends the action of ourselves and others and of all the persons and forces of the world. And this realisation can become absolute and complete in all the parts of our being only if we can have that sense and vision of it in all its forms, on all the levels of our being and the world being, as the material, vital, mental and supramental energy of the Divine, but all these, all the powers of all the planes must be seen and known as self-formulations of the one spiritual Shakti, infinite in being, consciousness and Ananda. It is not the invariable rule that this power should first manifest itself on the lower levels in the lower forms of energy and then reveal its higher spiritual nature. And if it does so come, first in its mental, vital or physical universalism, we must be careful not to rest content there. It may come instead at once in its higher reality, in the might of the spiritual splendour. The difficulty then will be to bear and hold the Power until it has laid powerful hands on and transformed the energies of the lower levels of the being. The difficulty will be less in proportion as we have been able to attain to a large quiet and equality, *samatā*, and either to realise, feel and live in the one tranquil immutable self in all or else to make a genuine and complete surrender of ourselves to the divine Master of the Yoga.

It is necessary here to keep always in mind the three powers of the Divine which are present and have to be taken account of in all living existences. In our ordinary consciousness we see these three as ourselves, the Jiva in the form of the ego, God—whatever conception we may have of God, and Nature. In the spiritual experience we see God as the supreme Self or Spirit, or as the Being from whom we come and in whom we live and move. We see Nature as his Power or God as Power, Spirit in Power acting in ourselves and the world. The Jiva is then himself this Self, Spirit, Divine, *so 'ham*, because he is one with him in essence of his being and consciousness, but as the individual he is only a portion of the Divine, a self of the Spirit, and in his natural being a form of the Shakti, a power of God in movement and action, *parā prakṛtir jīvabhūtā*. At first, when we become conscious of God or of the Shakti, the difficulties of our relation with them arise from the ego consciousness which we bring into the spiritual relation. The ego in us makes claims on the Divine other than the spiritual claim, and these claims are in a sense legitimate, but so long as and in proportion as they take the egoistic form, they are open to much grossness and great perversions, burdened with an element of falsehood, undesirable reaction and consequent evil, and the relation can only be wholly right, happy and perfect when these claims become part of the spiritual claim and lose their egoistic character. And in fact the claim of our being upon the Divine is fulfilled absolutely only then when it ceases at all to be a claim and is instead a fulfilment of the Divine through the individual, when we are satisfied with that alone, when we are content with the delight of oneness in being, content to leave the supreme Self and Master of existence to do whatever is the will of his absolute wisdom and knowledge through our more and more perfected Nature.

This is the sense of the self-surrender of the individual self to the Divine, *ātma-samarpaṇa*. It does not exclude a will for the delight of oneness, for participation in the divine consciousness, wisdom, knowledge, light, power, perfection, for the satisfaction of the divine fulfilment in us, but the will, the aspiration is ours because it is his will in us. At first, while there is still insistence on our own personality, it only reflects that, but becomes more and more indistinguishable from it, less personal and eventually it loses all shade of separateness, because the will in us has grown identical with the divine Tapas, the action of the divine Shakti.

And equally when we first become aware of the infinite Shakti above us or around or in us, the impulse of the egoistic sense in us is to lay hold on it and use this increased might for our egoistic purpose. This is a most dangerous thing, for it brings with it a sense and some increased reality of a great, sometimes a titanic power, and the rajasic ego, delighting in this sense of new enormous strength, may instead of waiting for it to be purified and transformed throw itself out in a violent and impure action and even turn us for a time or partially into the selfish and arrogant Asura using the strength given him for his own and not for the divine purpose: but on that way lies, in the end, if it is persisted in, spiritual perdition and material ruin. And even to regard oneself as the instrument of the Divine is not a perfect remedy; for when a strong ego meddles in the matter, it falsifies the spiritual relation and under cover of making itself an instrument of the Divine is really bent on making instead God its instrument. The one remedy is to still the egoistic claim of whatever kind, to lessen persistently the personal effort and individual straining which even the sattwic ego cannot avoid and instead of laying hold on the Shakti and using it for its purpose rather to let the Shakti lay hold on us and use us for the divine purpose. This cannot be done perfectly at once—nor can it be done safely if it is only the lower form of the universal energy of which we are aware, for then, as has already been said, there must be some other control, either of the mental Purusha or from above,—but still it is the aim which we must have before us and which can be wholly carried out when we become insistently aware of the highest spiritual presence and form of the divine Shakti. This surrender too of the whole action of the individual self to the Shakti is in fact a form of real self-surrender to the Divine.

It has been seen that a most effective way of purification is for the mental Purusha to draw back, to stand as the passive witness and observe and know himself and the workings of Nature in the lower, the normal being; but this must be combined, for perfection, with a will to raise the purified nature into the higher spiritual being. When that is done, the Purusha is no longer only a witness, but also the master of his prakriti, *īśvara*. At first it may not be apparent how this ideal of active self-mastery can be reconciled with the apparently opposite ideal of self-surrender and of becoming the assenting instrument of the divine Shakti. But in fact on the spiritual plane there is no difficulty. The Jiva cannot really become master except in proportion as he arrives at oneness with the Divine who is his supreme Self. And in that oneness and in his unity with the universe he is one too in the universal self with the will that directs all the operations of Nature. But more directly, less transcendentally, in his individual action too, he is a portion of the Divine and participates in the mastery over his nature of that to which he has surrendered himself. Even as instrument, he is not a mechanical but a conscious instrument. On the Purusha side of him he is one with the Divine and participates in the divine mastery of the Ishwara. On the nature side of him he is in his universality one with the power of the Divine, while in his individual natural being he is an instrument of the universal divine Shakti, because the individualised power is there to fulfil the purpose of the universal Power. The Jiva, as has been seen, is the meeting-place of the play of the dual aspect of the Divine, Prakriti and Purusha, and in the higher spiritual consciousness he becomes simultaneously one with both these aspects, and there he takes up and combines all the divine relations created by their interaction. This it is that makes possible the dual attitude.

There is however a possibility of arriving at this result without the passage through the passivity of the mental Purusha, by a more persistently and predominantly kinetic Yoga. Or there may be a combination of both the methods, alternations between them and an ultimate fusion. And here the problem of spiritual action assumes a more simple form. In this kinetic movement there are three stages. In the first the Jiva is aware of the supreme Shakti, receives the power into himself and uses it under her direction, with a certain sense of being the subordinate doer, a sense of minor responsibility in the action,—even at first, it may be, a responsibility for the result; but that disappears, for the result is seen to be determined by the higher Power, and only the action is felt to be partly his own. The sadhaka then feels that it is he who is thinking, willing, doing, but feels too the divine Shakti or Prakriti behind driving and shaping all his thought, will, feeling and action: the individual energy belongs in a way to him, but is still only a form and an instrument of the universal divine Energy. The Master of the Power may be hidden from him for a time by the action of the Shakti, or he may be aware of the Ishwara sometimes or continually manifest to him. In the latter case there are three things present to his consciousness, himself as the servant of the Ishwara, the Shakti behind as a great Power supplying the energy, shaping the action, formulating the results, the Ishwara above determining by his will the whole action.

In the second stage the individual doer disappears, but there is not necessarily any quietistic passivity; there may be a full kinetic action, only all is done by the Shakti. It is her power of knowledge which takes shape as thought in the mind; the sadhaka has no sense of himself thinking, but of the Shakti thinking in him. The will and the feelings and action are also in the same way nothing but a formation, operation, activity of the Shakti in her immediate presence and full possession of all the system. The sadhaka does not think, will, act, feel, but thought, will, feeling, action happen in his system. The individual on the side of action has disappeared into oneness with universal Prakriti, has become an individualised form and action of the divine Shakti. He is still aware of his personal existence, but it is as the Purusha supporting and observing the whole action, conscious of it in his self-knowledge and enabling by his participation the divine Shakti to do in him the works and the will of the Ishwara. The Master of the power is then sometimes hidden by the action of the power, sometimes appears governing it and compelling its workings. Here too there are three things present to the consciousness, the Shakti carrying on all the knowledge, thought, will, feeling, action for the Ishwara in an instrumental human form, the Ishwara, the Master of existence governing and compelling all her action, and ourself as the soul, the Purusha of her individual action enjoying all the relations with him which are created by her workings. There is another form of this realisation in which the Jiva disappears into and becomes one with the Shakti and there is then only the play of the Shakti with the Ishwara, Mahadeva and Kali, Krishna and Radha, the Deva and the Devi. This is the intensest possible form of the Jiva's realisation of himself as a manifestation of Nature, a power of the being of the Divine, *parā prakṛtir jīva-bhūtā*.

A third stage comes by the increasing manifestation of the Divine, the Ishwara in all our being and action. This is when we are constantly and uninterruptedly aware of him. He is felt in us as the possessor of our being and above us as the ruler of all its workings and they become to us nothing but a manifestation of him in the existence of the Jiva. All our consciousness is his consciousness, all our knowledge is his knowledge, all our thought is his thought, all our will is his will, all our feeling is his Ananda and form of his delight in being, all our action is his action. The distinction between the Shakti and the Ishwara begins to disappear; there is only the conscious activity in us of the Divine with the great self of the Divine behind and around and possessing it; all the world and Nature is seen to be only that, but here it has become fully conscious, the Maya of the ego removed, and the Jiva is there only as an eternal portion of his being, *aṁśa sanātana*, put forth to support a divine individualisation and living now fulfilled in the complete presence and power of the Divine, the complete joy of the Spirit manifested in the being. This is the highest realisation of the perfection and delight of the active oneness; for beyond it there could be only the consciousness of the Avatara, the Ishwara himself assuming a human name and form for action in the Lila.

# FAITH AND SHAKTI

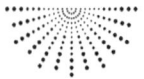

THE THREE parts of the perfection of our instrumental nature of which we have till now been reviewing the general features, the perfection of the intelligence, heart, vital consciousness and body, the perfection of the fundamental soul powers, the perfection of the surrender of our instruments and action to the divine Shakti, depend at every moment of their progression on a fourth power that is covertly and overtly the pivot of all endeavour and action, faith, *śraddhā*. The perfect faith is an assent of the whole being to the truth seen by it or offered to its acceptance, and its central working is a faith of the soul in its own will to be and attain and become and its idea of self and things and its knowledge, of which the belief of the intellect, the heart's consent and the desire of the life mind to possess and realise are the outward figures. This soul faith, in some form of itself, is indispensable to the action of the being and without it man cannot move a single pace in life, much less take any step forward to a yet unrealised perfection. It is so central and essential a thing that the Gita can justly say of it that whatever is a man's *śraddhā*, that he is, *yo yacchraddhaḥ sa eva saḥ*, and, it may be added, whatever he has the faith to see as possible in himself and strive for, that he can create and become. There is one kind of faith demanded as indispensable by the integral Yoga and that may be described as faith in God and the Shakti, faith in the presence and power of the Divine in us and the world, a faith that all in the world is the working of one divine Shakti, that all the steps of the Yoga, its strivings and sufferings and failures as well as its successes and satisfactions and victories are utilities and necessities of her workings and that by a firm and strong dependence on and a total self-surrender to the Divine and to his Shakti in us we can attain to oneness and freedom and victory and perfection.

The enemy of faith is doubt, and yet doubt too is a utility and necessity, because man in his ignorance and in his progressive labour towards knowledge needs to be visited by doubt, otherwise he would remain obstinate in an ignorant belief and limited knowledge and unable to escape from his errors. This utility and necessity of doubt does not altogether disappear when we enter on the path of Yoga. The integral Yoga aims at a knowledge not merely of some fundamental principle, but a knowing, a gnosis which will apply itself to and cover all life and the world action, and in this search for knowledge we enter on the way and are accompanied for many miles upon it by the mind's unregenerated activities before these are purified and transformed by a greater light: we carry with us a number of intellectual beliefs and ideas which are by no means all of them correct and perfect and a host of new ideas and suggestions meet us afterwards demanding our credence which it would be fatal to seize on and always cling to in the shape in which they come without regard to their possible error, limitation or imperfection. And indeed at one stage in the Yoga it becomes necessary to refuse to accept as definite and final any kind of intellectual idea or opinion whatever in its intellectual form and to hold it in a questioning suspension until it is given its right place and luminous shape of truth in a spiritual experience enlightened by supramental knowledge. And much more must this be the case with the desires or impulses of the life mind, which have often to be provisionally accepted as immediate indices of a temporarily necessary action before we have the full guidance, but not always clung to with the soul's complete assent, for eventually all these desires and impulses have to be rejected or else transformed into and replaced by impulses of the divine will taking up the life movements. The heart's faith, emotional beliefs, assents are also needed upon the way, but cannot be always sure guides until they too are taken up, purified, transformed and are eventually replaced by the luminous assents of a divine Ananda which is at one with the divine will and knowledge. In nothing in the lower nature from the reason to the vital will can the seeker of the Yoga put a complete and permanent faith, but only at last in the spiritual truth, power, Ananda which become in the spiritual reason his sole guides and luminaries and masters of action.

And yet faith is necessary throughout and at every step because it is a needed assent of the soul and without this assent there can be no progress. Our faith must first be abiding in the essential truth and principles of the Yoga, and even if this is clouded in the intellect, despondent in the heart, out-wearied and exhausted by constant denial and failure in the desire of the vital mind, there must be something in the innermost soul which clings and returns to it, otherwise we may fall on the path or abandon it from weakness and inability to bear temporary defeat, disappointment, difficulty and peril. In the Yoga as in life it is the man who persists unwearied to the last in the face of every defeat and disillusionment and of all confronting, hostile and contradicting events and powers who conquers in the end and finds his faith justified because to the soul and Shakti in man nothing is impossible. And even a blind and ignorant faith is a better possession than the sceptical doubt which turns its back on our spiritual possibilities or the constant carping of the narrow pettily critical uncreative intellect, *asū yā*, which pursues our endeavour with a paralysing incertitude. The seeker of the integral Yoga must however conquer both these imperfections. The thing to which he has given his assent and set his mind and heart and will to achieve, the divine perfection of the whole human being, is apparently an impossibility to the normal intelligence, since it is opposed to the actual facts of life and will for long be contradicted by immediate experience, as happens with all far-off and difficult ends, and it is denied too by many who have spiritual experience but believe that our present nature is the sole possible nature of man in the body and that it is only by throwing off the earthly life or even all individual existence that we can arrive at either a heavenly perfection or the release of extinction. In the pursuit of such an aim there will for long be plenty of ground for the objections, the carpings, *asūyā*, of that ignorant but persistent criticising reason which founds itself plausibly on the appearances of the moment, the stock of ascertained fact and experience, refuses to go beyond and questions the validity of all indices and illuminations that point forward; and if he yields to these narrow suggestions, he will either not arrive or be seriously hampered and long delayed in his journey. On the other hand ignorance and blindness in the faith are obstacles to a large success, invite much disappointment and disillusionment, fasten on false finalities and prevent advance to greater formulations of truth and perfection.

The Shakti in her workings will strike ruthlessly at all forms of ignorance and blindness and all even that trusts wrongly and superstitiously in her, and we must be prepared to abandon a too persistent attachment to forms of faith and cling to the saving reality alone. A great and wide spiritual and intelligent faith, intelligent with the intelligence of that larger reason which assents to high possibilities, is the character of the *śraddhā* needed for the integral Yoga.

This *śraddhā*—the English word faith is inadequate to express it—is in reality an influence from the supreme Spirit and its light a message from our supramental being which is calling the lower nature to rise out of its petty present to a great self-becoming and self-exceeding. And that which receives the influence and answers to the call is not so much the intellect, the heart or the life mind, but the inner soul which better knows the truth of its own destiny and mission. The circumstances that provoke our first entry into the path are not the real index of the thing that is at work in us. There the intellect, the heart, or the desires of the life mind may take a prominent place, or even more fortuitous accidents and outward incentives; but if these are all, then there can be no surety of our fidelity to the call and our enduring perseverance in the Yoga. The intellect may abandon the idea that attracted it, the heart weary or fail us, the desire of the life mind turn to other objectives. But outward circumstances are only a cover for the real workings of the spirit, and if it is the spirit that has been touched, the inward soul that has received the call, the *śraddhā* will remain firm and resist all attempts to defeat or slay it. It is not that the doubts of the intellect may not assail, the heart waver, the disappointed desire of the life mind sink down exhausted on the wayside. That is almost inevitable at times, perhaps often, especially with us, sons of an age of intellectuality and scepticism and a materialistic denial of spiritual truth which has not yet lifted its painted clouds from the face of the sun of a greater reality and is still opposed to the light of spiritual intuition and inmost experience. There will very possibly be many of those trying obscurations of which even the Vedic Rishis so often complained, "long exiles from the light", and these may be so thick, the night on the soul may be so black that faith may seem utterly to have left us. But through it all the spirit within will be keeping its unseen hold and the soul will return with a new strength to its assurance which was only eclipsed and not extinguished, because extinguished it cannot be when once the inner self has known and made its resolution.[1] The Divine holds our hand through all and if he seems to let us fall, it is only to raise us higher. This saving return we shall experience so often that the denials of doubt will become eventually impossible and, when once the foundation of equality is firmly established and still more when the sun of the gnosis has risen, doubt itself will pass away because its cause and utility have ended.

Moreover not only a faith in the fundamental principle, ideas, way of the Yoga is needed, but a day to day working faith in the power in us to achieve, in the steps we have taken on the way, in the spiritual experiences that come to us, in the intuitions, the guiding movements of will and impulsion, the moved intensities of the heart and aspirations and fulfilments of the life that are the aids, the circumstances and the stages of the enlarging of the nature and the stimuli or the steps of the soul's evolution. At the same time it has always to be remembered that we are moving from imperfection and ignorance towards light and perfection, and the faith in us must be free from attachment to the forms of our endeavour and the successive stages of our realisation. There is not only much that will be strongly raised in us in order to be cast out and rejected, a battle between the powers of ignorance and the lower nature and the higher powers that have to replace them, but experiences, states of thought and feeling, forms of realisation that are helpful and have to be accepted on the way and may seem to us for the time to be spiritual finalities, are found afterwards to be steps of transition, have to be exceeded and the working faith that supported them withdrawn in favour of other and greater things or of more full and comprehensive realisations and experiences, which replace them or into which they are taken up in a completing transformation. There can be for the seeker of the integral Yoga no clinging to resting-places on the road or to half-way houses; he cannot be satisfied till he has laid down all the great enduring bases of his perfection and broken out into its large and free infinities, and even there he has to be constantly filling himself with more experiences of the Infinite. His progress is an ascent from level to level and each new height brings in other vistas and revelations of the much that has still to be done, *bhūri kartvam*, till the divine Shakti has at last taken up all his endeavour and he has only to assent and participate gladly by a consenting oneness in her luminous workings. That which will support him through these changes, struggles, transformations which might otherwise dishearten and baffle,—for the intellect and life and emotion always grasp too much at things, fasten on premature certitudes and are apt to be afflicted and unwilling when forced to abandon that on which they rested,—is a firm faith in the Shakti that is at work and reliance on the guidance of the Master of the Yoga whose wisdom is not in haste and whose steps through all the perplexities of the mind are assured and just and sound, because they are founded on a perfectly comprehending transaction with the necessities of our nature.

The progress of the Yoga is a procession from the mental ignorance through imperfect formations to a perfect foundation and increasing of knowledge and in its more satisfyingly positive parts a movement from light to greater light, and it cannot cease till we have the greatest light of the supramental knowledge. The motions of the mind in its progress must necessarily be mixed with a greater or lesser proportion of error, and we should not allow our faith to be disconcerted by the discovery of its errors or imagine that because the beliefs of the intellect which aided us were too hasty and positive, therefore the fundamental faith in the soul was invalid. The human intellect is too much afraid of error precisely because it is too much attached to a premature sense of certitude and a too hasty eagerness for positive finality in what it seems to seize of knowledge. As our self-experience increases, we shall find that our errors even were necessary movements, brought with them and left their element or suggestion of truth and helped towards discovery or supported a necessary effort and that the certitudes we have now to abandon had yet their temporary validity in the progress of our knowledge. The intellect cannot be a sufficient guide in the search for spiritual truth and realisation and yet it has to be utilised in the integral movement of our nature. And while, therefore, we have to reject paralysing doubt or mere intellectual scepticism, the seeking intelligence has to be trained to admit a certain large questioning, an intellectual rectitude not satisfied with half-truths, mixtures of error or approximations and, most positive and helpful, a perfect readiness always to move forward from truths already held and accepted to the greater corrective, completing or transcending truths which at first it was unable or, it may be, disinclined to envisage. A working faith of the intellect is indispensable, not a superstitious, dogmatic or limiting credence attached to every temporary support or formula, but a large assent to the successive suggestions and steps of the Shakti, a faith fixed on realities, moving from the lesser to the completer realities and ready to throw down all scaffolding and keep only the large and growing structure.

A constant *śraddhā*, faith, assent of the heart and the life too are indispensable. But while we are in the lower nature the heart's assent is coloured by mental emotion and the life movements are accompanied by their trail of perturbing or straining desires, and mental emotion and desire tend to trouble, alter more or less grossly or subtly or distort the truth, and they always bring some limitation and imperfection into its realisation by the heart and life. The heart too when it is troubled in its attachments and its certitudes, perplexed by throw-backs and failures and convictions of error or involved in the wrestlings which attend a call to move forward from its assured positions, has its draggings, wearinesses, sorrowings, revolts, reluctances which hamper the progress. It must learn a larger and surer faith giving in the place of the mental reactions a calm or a moved spiritual acceptance to the ways and the steps of the Shakti which is in its nature the assent of a deepening Ananda to all necessary movements and a readiness to leave old moorings and move always forward towards the delight of a greater perfection. The life mind must give its assent to the successive motives, impulses, activities of the life imposed on it by the guiding power as aids or fields of the development of the nature and to the successions also of the inner Yoga, but it must not be attached or call a halt anywhere, but must always be prepared to abandon old urgency and accept with the same completeness of assent new higher movements and activities, and it must learn to replace desire by a wide and bright Ananda in all experience and action. The faith of the heart and the life mind, like that of the intelligence, must be capable of a constant correction, enlarging and transformation.

This faith is essentially the secret *śraddhā* of the soul, and it is brought more and more to the surface and there satisfied, sustained and increased by an increasing assurance and certainty of spiritual experience. Here too the faith in us must be unattached, a faith that waits upon Truth and is prepared to change and enlarge its understanding of spiritual experiences, to correct mistaken or half-true ideas about them and receive more enlightening interpretations, to replace insufficient by more sufficient intuitions, and to merge experiences that seemed at the time to be final and satisfying in more satisfying combinations with new experience and greater largenesses and transcendences. And especially in the psychical and other middle domains there is a very large room for the possibility of misleading and often captivating error, and here even a certain amount of positive scepticism has its use and at all events a great caution and scrupulous intellectual rectitude, but not the scepticism of the ordinary mind which amounts to a disabling denial. In the integral Yoga psychical experience, especially of the kind associated with what is often called occultism and savours of the miraculous, should be altogether subordinated to spiritual truth and wait upon that for its own interpretation, illumination and sanction. But even in the purely spiritual domain, there are experiences which are partial and, however attractive, only receive their full validity, significance or right application when we can advance to a fuller experience. And there are others which are in themselves quite valid and full and absolute, but if we confine ourselves to them, will prevent other sides of the spiritual truth from manifestation and mutilate the integrality of the Yoga. Thus the profound and absorbing quietude of impersonal peace which comes by the stilling of the mind is a thing in itself complete and absolute, but if we rest in that alone, it will exclude the companion absolute, not less great and needed and true, of the bliss of the divine action. Here too our faith must be an assent that receives all spiritual experience, but with a wide openness and readiness for always more light and truth, an absence of limiting attachment and no such clinging to forms as would interfere with the forward movement of the Shakti towards the integrality of the spiritual being, consciousness, knowledge, power, action and the wholeness of the one and the multiple Ananda.

The faith demanded of us both in its general principle and its constant particular application amounts to a large and ever increasing and a constantly purer, fuller and stronger assent of the whole being and all its parts to the presence and guidance of God and the Shakti. The faith in the Shakti, as long as we are not aware of and filled with her presence, must necessarily be preceded or at least accompanied by a firm and virile faith in our own spiritual will and energy and our power to move successfully towards unity and freedom and perfection. Man is given faith in himself, his ideas and his powers that he may work and create and rise to greater things and in the end bring his strength as a worthy offering to the altar of the Spirit. This spirit, says the Scripture, is not to be won by the weak, *nāyam ātmā balahīnena labhyaḥ*. All paralysing self-distrust has to be discouraged, all doubt of our strength to accomplish, for that is a false assent to impotence, an imagination of weakness and a denial of the omnipotence of the spirit. A present incapacity, however heavy may seem its pressure, is only a trial of faith and a temporary difficulty and to yield to the sense of inability is for the seeker of the integral Yoga a non-sense, for his object is a development of a perfection that is there already, latent in the being, because man carries the seed of the divine life in himself, in his own spirit, the possibility of success is involved and implied in the effort and victory is assured because behind is the call and guidance of an omnipotent power. At the same time this faith in oneself must be purified from all touch of rajasic egoism and spiritual pride. The sadhaka should keep as much as possible in his mind the idea that his strength is not his own in the egoistic sense but that of the divine universal Shakti and whatever is egoistic in his use of it must be a cause of limitation and in the end an obstacle.

The power of the divine universal Shakti which is behind our aspiration is illimitable, and when it is rightly called upon it cannot fail to pour itself into us and to remove whatever incapacity and obstacle, now or later; for the times and durations of our struggle while they depend at first, instrumentally and in part, on the strength of our faith and our endeavour, are yet eventually in the hands of the wisely determining secret Spirit, alone the Master of the Yoga, the Ishwara.

The faith in the divine Shakti must be always at the back of our strength and when she becomes manifest, it must be or grow implicit and complete. There is nothing that is impossible to her who is the conscious Power and universal Goddess all-creative from eternity and armed with the Spirit's omnipotence. All knowledge, all strengths, all triumph and victory, all skill and works are in her hands and they are full of the treasures of the Spirit and of all perfections and siddhis. She is Maheshwari, goddess of the supreme knowledge, and brings to us her vision for all kinds and widenesses of truth, her rectitude of the spiritual will, the calm and passion of her supramental largeness, her felicity of illumination: she is Mahakali, goddess of the supreme strength, and with her are all mights and spiritual force and severest austerity of tapas and swiftness to the battle and the victory and the laughter, the *aṭṭahāsya*, that makes light of defeat and death and the powers of the ignorance: she is Mahalakshmi, the goddess of the supreme love and delight, and her gifts are the spirit's grace and the charm and beauty of the Ananda and protection and every divine and human blessing: she is Mahasaraswati, the goddess of divine skill and of the works of the Spirit, and hers is the Yoga that is skill in works, *yogaḥ karmasu kauśalam*, and the utilities of divine knowledge and the self-application of the spirit to life and the happiness of its harmonies. And in all her powers and forms she carries with her the supreme sense of the masteries of the eternal Ishwari, a rapid and divine capacity for all kinds of action that may be demanded from the instrument, oneness, a participating sympathy, a free identity, with all energies in all beings and therefore a spontaneous and fruitful harmony with all the divine will in the universe. The intimate feeling of her presence and her powers and the satisfied assent of all our being to her workings in and around it is the last perfection of faith in the Shakti.

And behind her is the Ishwara and faith in him is the most central thing in the *śraddhā* of the integral Yoga. This faith we must have and develop to perfection that all things are the workings under the universal conditions of a supreme self-knowledge and wisdom, that nothing done in us or around us is in vain or without its appointed place and just significance, that all things are possible when the Ishwara as our supreme Self and Spirit takes up the action and that all that has been done before and all that he will do hereafter was and will be part of his infallible and foreseeing guidance and intended towards the fruition of our Yoga and our perfection and our life work. This faith will be more and more justified as the higher knowledge opens, we shall begin to see the great and small significances that escaped our limited mentality and faith will pass into knowledge. Then we shall see beyond the possibility of doubt that all happens within the working of the one Will and that that will was also wisdom because it develops always the true workings in life of the self and nature. The highest state of the assent, the *śraddhā* of the being will be when we feel the presence of the Ishwara and feel all our existence and consciousness and thought and will and action in his hand and consent in all things and with every part of our self and nature to the direct and immanent and occupying will of the Spirit. And that highest perfection of the *śraddhā* will also be the opportunity and perfect foundation of a divine strength: it will base, when complete, the development and manifestation and the works of the luminous supramental Shakti.

---

1. *saṅkalpa, vyavasāya.*

# THE NATURE OF THE SUPERMIND

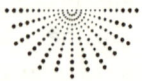

THE OBJECT of Yoga is to raise the human being from the consciousness of the ordinary mind subject to the control of vital and material Nature and limited wholly by birth and death and Time and the needs and desires of the mind, life and body to the consciousness of the spirit free in its self and using the circumstances of mind, life and body as admitted or self-chosen and self-figuring determinations of the spirit, using them in a free self-knowledge, a free will and power of being, a free delight of being. This is the essential difference between the ordinary mortal mind in which we live and the spiritual consciousness of our divine and immortal being which is the highest result of Yoga. It is a radical conversion as great as and greater than the change which we suppose evolutionary Nature to have made in its transition from the vital animal to the fully mentalised human consciousness. The animal has the conscious vital mind, but whatever beginnings there are in it of anything higher are only a primary glimpse, a crude hint of the intelligence which in man becomes the splendour of the mental understanding, will, emotion, aesthesis and reason. Man elevated in the heights and deepened by the intensities of the mind becomes aware of something great and divine in himself towards which all this tends, something he is in possibility but which he has not yet become, and he turns the powers of his mind, his power of knowledge, his power of will, his power of emotion and aesthesis to seek out this, to seize and comprehend all that it may be, to become it and to exist wholly in its greater consciousness, delight, being and power of highest becoming. But what he gets of this higher state in his normal mind is only an intimation, a primary glimpse, a crude hint of the splendour, the light, the glory and divinity of the spirit within him. A complete conversion of all the parts of his being into moulds and instruments of the spiritual consciousness is demanded of him before he can make quite real, constant, present to himself this greater thing that he can be and entirely live in what is now to him at the best a luminous aspiration. He must seek to develop and grow altogether into a greater divine consciousness by an integral Yoga.

The Yoga of perfection necessary to this change has, so far as we have been considering it, consisted in a preparatory purification of the mental, vital and physical nature, a liberation from the knots of the lower Prakriti, a consequent replacement of the egoistic state always subject to the ignorant and troubled action of the desire soul by a large and luminous static equality which quiets the reason, the emotional mind, the life mind and the physical nature and brings into us the peace and freedom of the spirit, and a dynamical substitution of the action of the supreme and universal divine Shakti under the control of the Ishwara for that of the lower Prakriti,—an action whose complete operation must be preceded by the perfection of the natural instruments. And all these things together, though not as yet the whole Yoga, constitute already a much greater than the present normal consciousness, spiritual in its basis and moved by a greater light, power and bliss, and it might be easy to rest satisfied with so much accomplished and think that all has been done that was needed for the divine conversion.

A momentous question however arises as light grows, the question through what medium is the divine Shakti to act in the human being? Is it to be always through the mind only and on the mind plane or in some greater supramental formulation which is more proper to a divine action and which will take up and replace the mental functions? If the mind is to be always the instrument, then although we shall be conscious of a diviner Power initiating and conducting all our inner and outer human action, yet it will have to formulate its knowledge, will, Ananda and all things else in the mental figure, and that means to translate them into an inferior kind of functioning other than the supreme workings native to the divine consciousness and its Shakti. The mind spiritualised, purified, liberated, perfected within its own limits may come as near as possible to a faithful mental translation, but we shall find that this is after all a relative fidelity and an imperfect perfection. The mind by its very nature cannot render with an entirely right rightness or act in the unified completeness of the divine knowledge, will and Ananda because it is an instrument for dealing with the divisions of the finite on the basis of division, a secondary instrument therefore and a sort of delegate for the lower movement in which we live. The mind can reflect the Infinite, it can dissolve itself into it, it can live in it by a large passivity, it can take its suggestions and act them out in its own way, a way always fragmentary, derivative and subject to a greater or less deformation, but it cannot be itself the direct and perfect instrument of the infinite Spirit acting in its own knowledge. The divine Will and Wisdom organising the action of the infinite consciousness and determining all things according to the truth of the spirit and the law of its manifestation is not mental but supramental and even in its formulation nearest to mind as much above the mental consciousness in its light and power as the mental consciousness of man above the vital mind of the lower creation. The question is how far the perfected human being can raise himself above mind, enter into some kind of fusing union with the supramental and build up in himself a level of supermind, a developed gnosis by the form and power of which the divine Shakti can directly act, not through a mental translation, but organically in her supramental nature.

It is here necessary in a matter so remote from the ordinary lines of our thought and experience to state first what is the universal gnosis or divine supermind, how it is represented in the actual movement of the universe and what are its relations to the present psychology of the human being. It will then be evident that though the supermind is supra-rational to our intelligence and its workings occult to our apprehension, it is nothing irrationally mystic, but rather its existence and emergence is a logical necessity of the nature of existence, always provided we grant that not matter or mind alone but spirit is the fundamental reality and everywhere a universal presence. All things are a manifestation of the infinite spirit out of its own being, out of its own consciousness and by the self-realising, self-determining, self-fulfilling power of that consciousness. The Infinite, we may say, organises by the power of its self-knowledge the law of its own manifestation of being in the universe, not only the material universe present to our senses, but whatever lies behind it on whatever planes of existence. All is organised by it not under any inconscient compulsion, not according to a mental fantasy or caprice, but in its own infinite spiritual freedom according to the self-truth of its being, its infinite potentialities and its will of self-creation out of those potentialities, and the law of this self-truth is the necessity that compels created things to act and evolve each according to its own nature. The Intelligence—to give it an inadequate name—the Logos that thus organises its own manifestation is evidently something infinitely greater, more extended in knowledge, compelling in self-power, large both in the delight of its self-existence and the delight of its active being and works than the mental intelligence which is to us the highest realised degree and expression of consciousness. It is to this intelligence infinite in itself but freely organising and self-determiningly organic in its self-creation and its works that we may give for our present purpose the name of the divine supermind or gnosis.

The fundamental nature of this supermind is that all its knowledge is originally a knowledge by identity and oneness and even when it makes numberless apparent divisions and discriminating modifications in itself, still all the knowledge that operates in its workings, even in these divisions, is founded upon and sustained and lit and guided by this perfect knowledge by identity and oneness. The Spirit is one everywhere and it knows all things as itself and in itself, so sees them always and therefore knows them intimately, completely, in their reality as well as their appearance, in their truth, their law, the entire spirit and sense and figure of their nature and their workings. When it sees anything as an object of knowledge, it yet sees it as itself and in itself, and not as a thing other than or divided from it about which therefore it would at first be ignorant of the nature, constitution and workings and have to learn about them, as the mind is at first ignorant of its object and has to learn about it because the mind is separated from its object and regards and senses and meets it as something other than itself and external to its own being. The mental awareness we have of our own subjective existence and its movements, though it may point to, is not the same thing as this identity and self-knowledge, because what it sees are mental figures of our being and not the inmost or the whole and it is only a partial, derivative and superficial action of our self that appears to us while the largest and most secretly determining parts of our own existence are occult to our mentality. The supramental Spirit has, unlike the mental being, the real because the inmost and total knowledge of itself and of all its universe and of all things that are its creations and self-figurings in the universe.

This is the second character of the supreme Supermind that its knowledge is a real because a total knowledge. It has in the first place a transcendental vision and sees the universe not only in the universal terms, but in its right relation to the supreme and eternal reality from which it proceeds and of which it is an expression. It knows the spirit and truth and whole sense of the universal expression because it knows all the essentiality and all the infinite reality and all the consequent constant potentiality of that which in part it expresses. It knows rightly the relative because it knows the Absolute and all its absolutes to which the relatives refer back and of which they are the partial or modified or suppressed figures. It is in the second place universal and sees all that is individual in the terms of the universal as well as in its own individual terms and holds all these individual figures in their right and complete relation to the universe. It is in the third place, separately with regard to individual things, total in its view because it knows each in its inmost essence of which all else is the resultant, in its totality which is its complete figure and in its parts and their connections and dependences, —as well as in its connections with and its dependences upon other things and its nexus with the total implications and the explicits of the universe.

The mind on the contrary is limited and incapable in all these directions. Mind cannot arrive at identity with the Absolute even when by a stretch of the intellect it conceives the idea, but can only disappear into it in a swoon or extinction: it can only have a kind of sense or an intimation of certain absolutes which it puts by the mental idea into a relative figure. It cannot grasp the universal, but only arrives at some idea of it through an extension of the individual or a combination of apparently separate things and so sees it either as a vague infinite or indeterminate or a half-determined largeness or else only in an external scheme or constructed figure. The indivisible being and action of the universal, which is its real truth, escapes the apprehension of the mind, because the mind thinks it out analytically by taking its own divisions for units and synthetically by combinations of these units, but cannot seize on and think entirely in the terms, though it may get at the idea and certain secondary results, of the essential oneness. It cannot, either, know truly and thoroughly even the individual and apparently separate thing, because it proceeds in the same way, by an analysis of parts and constituents and properties and a combination by which it erects a scheme of it which is only its external figure. It can get an intimation of the essential inmost truth of its object, but cannot live constantly and luminously in that essential knowledge and work out on the rest from within outward so that the outward circumstances appear in their intimate reality and meaning as inevitable result and expression and form and action of the spiritual something which is the reality of the object. And all this which is impossible for the mind to do, but possible only to strive towards and figure, is inherent and natural to the supramental knowledge.

The third characteristic of the supermind arising from this difference, which brings us to the practical distinction between the two kinds of knowledge, is that it is directly truth-conscious, a divine power of immediate, inherent and spontaneous knowledge, an Idea holding luminously all realities and not depending on indications and logical or other steps from the known to the unknown like the mind which is a power of the Ignorance. The supermind contains all its knowledge in itself, is in its highest divine wisdom in eternal possession of all truth and even in its lower, limited or individualised forms has only to bring the latent truth out of itself,—the perception which the old thinkers tried to express when they said that all knowing was in its real origin and nature only a memory of inwardly existing knowledge. The supermind is eternally and on all levels truth-conscious and exists secretly even in mental and material being, surveys and knows the things, even obscurest, of the mental ignorance and understands and is behind and governs its processes, because everything in the mind derives from the supermind—and must do so because everything derives from the spirit. All that is mental is but a partial, a modified, a suppressed or half-suppressed figure of the supramental truth, a deformation or a derived and imperfect figure of its greater knowledge. The mind begins with ignorance and proceeds towards knowledge. As an actual fact, in the material universe, it appears out of an initial and universal inconscience which is really an involution of the all-conscient spirit in its own absorbed self-oblivious force of action; and it appears therefore as part of an evolutionary process, first a vital feeling towards overt sensation, then an emergence of a vital mind capable of sensation and, evolving out of it, a mind of emotion and desire, a conscious will, a growing intelligence. And each stage is an emergence of a greater suppressed power of the secret supermind and spirit.

The mind of man, capable of reflection and a coordinated investigation and understanding of itself and its basis and surroundings, arrives at truth but against a background of original ignorance, a truth distressed by a constant surrounding mist of incertitude and error. Its certitudes are relative and for the most part precarious certainties or else are the assured fragmentary certitudes only of an imperfect, incomplete and not an essential experience. It makes discovery after discovery, gets idea after idea, adds experience to experience and experiment to experiment,—but losing and rejecting and forgetting and having to recover much as it proceeds,—and it tries to establish a relation between all that it knows by setting up logical and other sequences, a series of principles and their dependences, generalisations and their application, and makes out of its devices a structure in which mentally it can live, move and act and enjoy and labour. This mental knowledge is always limited in extent: not only so, but in addition the mind even sets up other willed barriers, admitting by the mental device of opinion certain parts and sides of truth and excluding all the rest, because if it gave free admission and play to all ideas, if it suffered truth's infinities, it would lose itself in an unreconciled variety, an undetermined immensity and would be unable to act and proceed to practical consequences and an effective creation. And even when it is widest and most complete, mental knowing is still an indirect knowledge, a knowledge not of the thing in itself but of its figures, a system of representations, a scheme of indices,—except indeed when in certain movements it goes beyond itself, beyond the mental idea to spiritual identity, but it finds it extremely difficult to go here beyond a few isolated and intense spiritual realisations or to draw or work out or organise the right practical consequences of these rare identities of knowledge. A greater power than the reason is needed for the spiritual comprehension and effectuation of this deepest knowledge.

This is what the supermind, intimate with the Infinite, alone can do. The supermind sees directly the spirit and essence, the face and body, the result and action, the principles and dependences of the truth as one indivisible whole and therefore can work out the circumstantial results in the power of the essential knowledge, the variations of the spirit in the light of its identities, its apparent divisions in the truth of its oneness. The supermind is a knower and creator of its own truth, the mind of man only a knower and creator in the half light and half darkness of a mingled truth and error, and creator too of a thing which it derives altered, translated, lessened from something greater than and beyond it. Man lives in a mental consciousness between a vast subconscient which is to his seeing a dark inconscience and a vaster superconscient which he is apt to take for another but a luminous inconscience, because his idea of consciousness is confined to his own middle term of mental sensation and intelligence. It is in that luminous superconscience that there lie the ranges of the supermind and the spirit.

The supermind is again, because it acts and creates as well as knows, not only a direct truth-consciousness, but an illumined, direct and spontaneous truth-will. There is not and cannot be in the will of the self-knowing spirit any contradiction, division or difference between its will and its knowledge. The spiritual will is the Tapas or enlightened force of the conscious being of the spirit effecting infallibly what is there within it, and it is this infallible operation of things acting according to their own nature, of energy producing result and event according to the force within it, of action bearing the fruit and event involved in its own character and intention which we call variously in its different aspects law of Nature, Karma, Necessity and Fate. These things are to mind the workings of a power outside or above it in which it is involved and intervenes only with a contributory personal effort which partly arrives and succeeds, partly fails and stumbles and which even in succeeding is largely overruled for issues different from or at any rate greater and more far-reaching than its own intention. The will of man works in the ignorance by a partial light or more often flickerings of light which mislead as much as they illuminate. His mind is an ignorance striving to erect standards of knowledge, his will an ignorance striving to erect standards of right, and his whole mentality as a result very much a house divided against itself, idea in conflict with idea, the will often in conflict with the ideal of right or the intellectual knowledge. The will itself takes different shapes, the will of the intelligence, the wishes of the emotional mind, the desires and the passion of the vital being, the impulsions and blind or half-blind compulsions of the nervous and the subconscient nature, and all these make by no means a harmony, but at best a precarious concord among discords. The will of the mind and life is a stumbling about in search of right force, right Tapas which can wholly be attained in its true and complete light and direction only by oneness with the spiritual and supramental being.

The supramental nature on the contrary is just, harmonious and one, will and knowledge there only light of the spirit and power of the spirit, the power effecting the light, the light illuming the power. In the highest supramentality they are intimately fused together and do not even wait upon each other but are one movement, will illumining itself, knowledge fulfilling itself, both together a single jet of the being. The mind knows only the present and lives in an isolated movement of it though it tries to remember and retain the past and forecast and compel the future. The supermind has the vision of the three times, *trikāladṛṣṭi*; it sees them as an indivisible movement and sees too each containing the others. It is aware of all tendencies, energies and forces as the diverse play of unity and knows their relation to each other in the single movement of the one spirit. The supramental will and action are therefore a will and action of the spontaneous self-fulfilling truth of the spirit, the right and at the highest the infallible movement of a direct and total knowledge.

The supreme and universal Supermind is the active Light and Tapas of the supreme and universal Self as the Lord and Creator, that which we come to know in Yoga as the divine Wisdom and Power, the eternal knowledge and will of the Ishwara. On the highest planes of Being where all is known and all manifests as existences of the one existence, consciousnesses of the one consciousness, delight's self-creations of the one Ananda, many truths and powers of the one Truth, there is the intact and integral display of its spiritual and supramental knowledge. And in the corresponding planes of our own being the Jiva shares in the spiritual and supramental nature and lives in its light and power and bliss. As we descend nearer to what we are in this world, the presence and action of this self-knowledge narrows but retains always the essence and character when not the fullness of the supramental nature and its way of knowing and willing and acting, because it still lives in the essence and body of the spirit. The mind, when we trace the descent of the self towards matter, we see as a derivation which travels away from the fullness of self, the fullness of its light and being and which lives in a division and diversion, not in the body of the sun, but first in its nearer and then in its far-off rays. There is a highest intuitive mind which receives more nearly the supramental truth, but even this is a formation which conceals the direct and greater real knowledge. There is an intellectual mind which is a luminous half-opaque lid which intercepts and reflects in a radiantly distorting and suppressively modifying atmosphere the truth known to the supermind. There is a still lower mind built on the foundation of the senses between which and the sun of knowledge there is a thick cloud, an emotional and a sensational mist and vapour with here and there lightnings and illuminations. There is a vital mind which is shut away even from the light of intellectual truth, and lower still in submental life and matter the spirit involves itself entirely as if in a sleep and a night, a sleep plunged in a dim and yet poignant nervous dream, the night of a mechanical somnambulist energy. It is a re-evolution of the spirit out of this lowest state in which we find ourselves at a height above the lower creation having taken it up all in us and reaching so far in our ascent only the light of the well-developed mental reason. The full powers of self-knowledge and the illumined will of the spirit are still beyond us above the mind and reason in supramental Nature.

If the spirit is everywhere, even in matter—in fact matter itself is only an obscure form of the spirit—and if the supermind is the universal power of the spirit's omnipresent self-knowledge organising all the manifestation of the being, then in matter and everywhere there must be present a supramental action and, however concealed it may be by another, lower and obscurer kind of operation, yet when we look close we shall find that it is really the supermind which organises matter, life, mind and reason. And this actually is the knowledge towards which we are now moving. There is even a quite visible intimate action of the consciousness, persistent in life, matter and mind, which is clearly a supramental action subdued to the character and need of the lower medium and to which we now give the name of intuition from its most evident characteristics of direct vision and self-acting knowledge, really a vision born of some secret identity with the object of the knowledge. What we call the intuition is however only a partial indication of the presence of the supermind, and if we take this presence and power in its widest character, we shall see that it is a concealed supramental force with a self-conscious knowledge in it which informs the whole action of material energy. It is that which determines what we call law of nature, maintains the action of each thing according to its own nature and harmonises and evolves the whole, which would otherwise be a fortuitous creation apt at any moment to collapse into chaos. All the law of nature is a thing precise in its necessities of process, but is yet in the cause of that necessity and of its constancy of rule, measure, combination, adaptation, result a thing inexplicable, meeting us at every step with a mystery and a miracle, and this must be either because it is irrational and accidental even in its regularities or because it is suprarational, because the truth of it belongs to a principle greater than that of our intelligence. That principle is the supramental; that is to say, the hidden secret of Nature is the organisation of something out of the infinite potentialities of the self-existent truth of the spirit the nature of which is wholly evident only to an original knowledge born of and proceeding by a fundamental identity, the spirit's constant self-perception. All the action of life too is of this character and all the action of mind and reason,—reason which is the first to perceive everywhere the action of a greater reason and law of being and try to render it by its own conceptional structures, though it does not always perceive that it is something other than a mental Intelligence which is at work, other than an intellectual Logos. All these processes are actually spiritual and supramental in their secret government, but mental, vital and physical in their overt process.

The outward matter, life, mind do not possess this occult action of the supermind, even while possessed and compelled by the necessity it imposes on their workings. There is what we are sometimes moved to call an intelligence and will operating in the material force and the atom (although the words ring false because it is not actually the same thing as our own will and intelligence),—let us say, a covert intuition of self-existence at work,—but the atom and force are not aware of it and are only the obscure body of matter and of power created by its first effort of self-manifestation. The presence of such an intuition becomes more evident to us in all the action of life because that is nearer to our own scale. And as life develops overt sense and mind, as in the animal creation, we can speak more confidently of a vital intuition which is behind its operations and which emerges in the animal mind in the clear form of instinct,—instinct, an automatic knowledge implanted in the animal, sure, direct, self-existent, self-guided, which implies somewhere in its being an accurate knowing of purpose, relation and the thing or object. It acts in the life force and mind, but yet the surface life and mind do not possess it and cannot give an account of what it does or control or extend the power at its will and pleasure. Here we observe two things, first, that the overt intuition acts only for a limited necessity and purpose, and that in the rest of the operations of the nature there is a double action, one uncertain and ignorant of the surface consciousness and the other subliminal implying a secret subconscient direction. The surface consciousness is full of a groping and seeking which increases rather than diminishes as life rises in its scale and widens in the scope of its conscious powers; but the secret self within assures in spite of the groping of the vital mind the action of the nature and the result needed for the necessity, the purpose and the destiny of the being. This continues on a higher and higher scale up to the human reason and intelligence.

The being of man also is full of physical, vital, emotional, psychical and dynamic instincts and intuitions, but he does not rely on them as the animal does,—though they are capable in him of a far larger scope and greater action than in the animal and lower creation by reason of his greater actual evolutionary development and his yet greater potentiality of development of the being. He has suppressed them, discontinued their full and overt action by atrophy,—not that these capacities are destroyed but rather held back or cast back into the subliminal consciousness,—and consequently this lower part of his being is much less sure of itself, much less confident of the directions of his nature, much more groping, errant and fallible in its larger scope than that of the animal in his lesser limits. This happens because man's real dharma and law of being is to seek for a greater self-aware existence, a self-manifestation no longer obscure and governed by an ununderstood necessity, but illumined, conscious of that which is expressing itself and able to give it a fuller and more perfect expression. And finally his culmination must be to identify himself with his greatest and real self and act or rather let it act (his natural existence being an instrumental form of the expression of the spirit) in its spontaneous perfect will and knowledge. His first instrument for this transition is the reason and the will of the rational intelligence and he is moved to depend upon that to the extent of its development for his knowledge and guidance and give it the control of the rest of his being. And if the reason were the highest thing and the greatest all-sufficient means of the self and spirit, he could by it know perfectly and guide perfectly all the movements of his nature. This he cannot do entirely because his self is a larger thing than his reason and if he limits himself by the rational will and intelligence, he imposes an arbitrary restriction both in extent and in kind on his self-development, self-expression, knowledge, action, Ananda. The other parts of his being demand too a complete expression in the largeness and perfection of the self and cannot have it if their expression is changed in kind and carved, cut down and arbitrarily shaped and mechanised in action by the inflexible machinery of the rational intelligence. The godhead of the reason, the intellectual Logos, is only a partial representative and substitute for the greater supramental Logos, and its function is to impose a preliminary partial knowledge and order upon the life of the creature, but the real, final and integral order can only be founded by the spiritual supermind in its emergence.

The supermind in the lower nature is present most strongly as intuition and it is therefore by a development of an intuitive mind that we can make the first step towards the self-existent spontaneous and direct supramental knowledge. All the physical, vital, emotional, psychic, dynamic nature of man is a surface seizing of suggestions which rise out of a subliminal intuitive self-being of these parts, and an attempt usually groping and often circuitous to work them out in the action of a superficial embodiment and power of the nature which is not overtly enlightened by the inner power and knowledge. An increasingly intuitive mind has the best chance of discovering what they are seeking for and leading them to the desired perfection of their self-expression. The reason itself is only a special kind of application, made by a surface regulating intelligence, of suggestions which actually come from a concealed, but sometimes partially overt and active power of the intuitive spirit. In all its action there is at the covered or half-covered point of origination something which is not the creation of the reason, but given to it either directly by the intuition or indirectly through some other part of the mind for it to shape into intellectual form and process. The rational judgment in its decisions and the mechanical process of the logical intelligence, whether in its more summary or in its more developed operations, conceals while it develops the true origin and native substance of our will and thinking. The greatest minds are those in which this veil wears thin and there is the largest part of intuitive thinking, which often no doubt but not always brings with it a great accompanying display of intellectual action. The intuitive intelligence is however never quite pure and complete in the present mind of man, because it works in the medium of mind and is at once seized on and coated over with a mixed stuff of mentality. It is as yet not brought out, not developed and perfected so as to be sufficient for all the operations now performed by the other mental instruments, not trained to take them up and change them into or replace them by its own fullest, most direct, assured and sufficient workings. This can indeed only be done if we make the intuitive mind a transitional means for bringing out the secret supermind itself of which it is a mental figure and forming in our frontal consciousness a body and instrument of supermind which will make it possible for the self and spirit to display itself in its own largeness and splendour.

    It must be remembered that there is always a difference between the supreme Supermind of the omniscient and omnipotent Ishwara and that which can be attained by the Jiva. The human being is climbing out of the ignorance and when he ascends into the supramental nature, he will find in it grades of its ascension, and he must first form the lower grades and limited steps before he rises to higher summits. He will enjoy there the full essential light, power, Ananda of the infinite self by oneness with the Spirit, but in the dynamical expression it must determine and individualise itself according to the nature of the self-expression which the transcendent and universal Spirit seeks in the Jiva. It is God-realisation and God-expression which is the object of our Yoga and more especially of its dynamic side, it is a divine self-expression in us of the Ishwara, but under the conditions of humanity and through the divinised human nature.

# THE INTUITIVE MIND

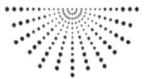

THE ORIGINAL nature of supermind is the self-conscience and all-conscience of the Infinite, of the universal Spirit and Self in things, organising on the foundation and according to the character of a direct self-knowledge its own wisdom and effective omnipotence for the unfolding and the regulated action of the universe and of all things in the universe. It is, we might say, the gnosis of the Spirit master of its own cosmos, *ātmā jñātā īśvaraḥ*. As it knows itself, so too it knows all things—for all are only becomings of itself—directly, totally and from within outward, spontaneously in detail and arrangement, each thing in the truth of itself and its nature and in its relation to all other things. And it knows similarly all action of its energy in antecedent or cause and occasion of manifestation and effect or consequence, all things in infinite and in limited potentiality and in selection of actuality and in their succession of past, present and future. The organising supermind of a divine being in the universe would be a delegation of this omnipotence and omniscience for the purpose and within the scope of his own action and nature and of all that comes into its province. The supermind in an individual would be a similar delegation on whatever scale and within whatever province. But while in the god this would be a direct and an immediate delegation of a power illimitable in itself and limited only in action, but otherwise unaltered in operation, natural to the being and full and free always, in man any emergence of the supermind must be a gradual and at first an imperfect creation and to his customary mind the activity of an exceptional and supernormal will and knowledge.

In the first place it will not be for him a native power always enjoyed without interruption, but a secret potentiality which has to be discovered and one for which there are no organs in his present physical or mental system: he has either to evolve a new organ for it or else to adopt or transform existing ones and make them utilisable for the purpose. He has not merely to uncover the hidden sun of the supermind in the subliminal cavern of his secret being or remove the cloud of his mental ignorance from its face in the spiritual skies so that it shall at once shine out in all its glory. His task is much more complex and difficult because he is an evolutionary being and by the evolution of Nature of which he is a part he has been constituted with an inferior kind of knowledge, and this inferior, this mental power of knowledge forms by its persistent customary action an obstacle to a new formation greater than its own nature. A limited mental intelligence enlightening a limited mind of sense and the capacity not always well used of a considerable extension of it by the use of the reason are the powers by which he is at present distinguished from all other terrestrial creatures. This sense mind, this intelligence, this reason, however inadequate, are the instruments in which he has learned to put his trust and he has erected by their means certain foundations which he is not over willing to disturb and has traced limits outside of which he feels all to be confusion, uncertainty and a perilous adventure. Moreover the transition to the higher principle means not only a difficult conversion of his whole mind and reason and intelligence, but in a certain sense a reversal of all their methods. The soul climbing above a certain critical line of change sees all its former operations as an inferior and ignorant action and has to effect another kind of working which sets out from a different starting-point and has quite another kind of initiation of the energy of the being. If an animal mind were called upon to leave consciently the safe ground of sense impulse, sense understanding and instinct for the perilous adventure of a reasoning intelligence, it might well turn back alarmed and unwilling from the effort. The human mind would here be called upon to make a still greater change and, although self-conscious and adventurous in the circle of its possibility, might well hold this to be beyond the circle and reject the adventure. In fact the change is only possible if there is first a spiritual development on our present level of consciousness and it can only be undertaken securely when the mind has become aware of the greater self within, enamoured of the Infinite and confident of the presence and guidance of the Divine and his Shakti.

The problem of this conversion resolves itself at first into a passage through a mediary status and by the help of the one power already at work in the human mind which we can recognise as something supramental in its nature or at least in its origin, the faculty of intuition, a power of which we can feel the presence and the workings and are impressed, when it acts, by its superior efficiency, light, direct inspiration and force, but cannot understand or analyse it as we understand or analyse the workings of our reason. The reason understands itself, but not what is beyond it,—of that it can only make a general figure or representation; the supermind alone can discern the method of its own workings. The power of intuition acts in us at present for the most part in a covert manner secret and involved in or mostly veiled by the action of the reason and the normal intelligence; so far as it emerges into a clear separate action, it is still occasional, partial, fragmentary and of an intermittent character. It casts a sudden light, it makes a luminous suggestion or it throws out a solitary brilliant clue or scatters a small number of isolated or related intuitions, lustrous discriminations, inspirations or revelations, and it leaves the reason, will, mental sense or intelligence to do what each can or pleases with this seed of succour that has come to them from the depths or the heights of our being. The mental powers immediately proceed to lay hold on these things and to manipulate and utilise them for our mental or vital purposes, to adapt them to the forms of the inferior knowledge, to coat them up in or infiltrate them with the mental stuff and suggestion, often altering their truth in the process and always limiting their potential force of enlightenment by these accretions and by this subdual to the exigencies of the inferior agent, and almost always they make at once too little and too much of them, too little by not allowing them time to settle and extend their full power for illumination, too much by insisting on them or rather on the form into which the mentality casts them to the exclusion of the larger truth that the more consistent use of the intuitive faculty might have given. Thus the intuition intervening in the ordinary mental operations acts in lightning flashes that make lustrous a space of truth, but is not a steady sunlight illumining securely the whole reach and kingdom of our thought and will and feeling and action.

It appears at once that there are two necessary lines of progress which we must follow, and the first is to extend the action of the intuition and make it more constant, more persistent and regular and all-embracing until it is so intimate and normal to our being that it can take up all the action now done by the ordinary mind and assume its place in the whole system. This cannot wholly be done so long as the ordinary mind continues to assert its power of independent action and intervention or its habit of seizing on the light of the intuition and manipulating it for its own purposes. The higher mentality cannot be complete or secure so long as the inferior intelligence is able to deform it or even to bring in any of its own intermixture. And either then we must silence altogether the intellect and the intellectual will and the other inferior activities and leave room only for the intuitive action or we must lay hold on and transform the lower action by the constant pressure of the intuition. Or else there must be an alternation and combination of the two methods if that be the most natural way or at all possible. The actual process and experience of Yoga manifests the possibility of several methods or movements none of which by itself produces the entire result in practice, however it may seem at first sight that logically each should or might be adequate. And when we learn to insist on no particular method as exclusively the right one and leave the whole movement to a greater guidance, we find that the divine Lord of the Yoga commissions his Shakti to use one or the other at different times and all in combination according to the need and turn of the being and the nature.

At first it might seem the straight and right way to silence the mind altogether, to silence the intellect, the mental and personal will, the desire mind and the mind of emotion and sensation, and to allow in that perfect silence the Self, the Spirit, the Divine to disclose himself and leave him to illuminate the being by the supramental light and power and Ananda. And this is indeed a great and powerful discipline. It is the calm and still mind much more readily and with a much greater purity than the mind in agitation and action that opens to the Infinite, reflects the Spirit, becomes full of the Self and awaits like a consecrated and purified temple the unveiling of the Lord of all our being and nature. It is true also that the freedom of this silence gives a possibility of a larger play of the intuitive being and admits with less obstruction and turmoil of mental groping and seizing the great intuitions, inspirations, revelations which emerge from within or descend from above. It is therefore an immense gain if we can acquire the capacity of always being able at will to command an absolute tranquillity and silence of the mind free from any necessity of mental thought or movement and disturbance and, based in that silence, allow thought and will and feeling to happen in us only when the Shakti wills it and when it is needful for the divine purpose. It becomes easier then to change the manner and character of the thought and will and feeling. Nevertheless it is not the fact that by this method the supramental light will immediately replace the lower mind and reflective reason. When the inner action proceeds after the silence, even if it be then a more predominatingly intuitive thought and movement, the old powers will yet interfere, if not from within, then by a hundred suggestions from without, and an inferior mentality will mix in, will question or obstruct or will try to lay hold on the greater movement and to lower or darken or distort or minimise it in the process. Therefore the necessity of a process of elimination or transformation of the inferior mentality remains always imperative,—or perhaps both at once, an elimination of all that is native to the lower being, its disfiguring accidents, its depreciations of value, its distortions of substance and all else that the greater truth cannot harbour, and a transformation of the essential things our mind derives from the supermind and spirit but represents in the manner of the mental ignorance.

A second movement is one which comes naturally to those who commence the Yoga with the initiative that is proper to the way of Bhakti. It is natural to them to reject the intellect and its action and to listen for the voice, wait for the impulsion or the command, the *ādeśa*, obey only the idea and will and power of the Lord within them, the divine Self and Purusha in the heart of the creature, *īśvaraḥ sarvabhūtānāṁ hṛddeśe*. This is a movement which must tend more and more to intuitivise the whole nature, for the ideas, the will, the impulsions, the feelings which come from the secret Purusha in the heart are of the direct intuitive character. This method is consonant with a certain truth of our nature. The secret Self within us is an intuitive self and this intuitive self is seated in every centre of our being, the physical, the nervous, the emotional, the volitional, the conceptual or cognitive and the higher more directly spiritual centres. And in each part of our being it exercises a secret intuitive initiation of our activities which is received and represented imperfectly by our outer mind and converted into the movements of the ignorance in the external action of these parts of our nature. The heart or emotional centre of the thinking desire mind is the strongest in the ordinary man, gathers up or at least affects the presentation of things to the consciousness and is the capital of the system. It is from there that the Lord seated in the heart of all creatures turns them mounted on the machine of Nature by the Maya of the mental ignorance. It is possible then by referring back all the initiation of our action to this secret intuitive Self and Spirit, the ever-present Godhead within us, and replacing by its influences the initiations of our personal and mental nature to get back from the inferior external thought and action to another, internal and intuitive, of a highly spiritualised character. Nevertheless the result of this movement cannot be complete, because the heart is not the highest centre of our being, is not supramental nor directly moved from the supramental sources. An intuitive thought and action directed from it may be very luminous and intense but is likely to be limited, even narrow in its intensity, mixed with a lower emotional action and at the best excited and troubled, rendered unbalanced or exaggerated by a miraculous or abnormal character in its action or at least in many of its accompaniments which is injurious to the harmonised perfection of the being. The aim of our effort at perfection must be to make the spiritual and supramental action no longer a miracle, even if a frequent or constant miracle, or only a luminous intervention of a greater than our natural power, but normal to the being and the very nature and law of all its process.

The highest organised centre of our embodied being and of its action in the body is the supreme mental centre figured by the yogic symbol of the thousand-petalled lotus, *sahasradala*, and it is at its top and summit that there is the direct communication with the supramental levels. It is then possible to adopt a different and a more direct method, not to refer all our thought and action to the Lord secret in the heart-lotus but to the veiled truth of the Divinity above the mind and to receive all by a sort of descent from above, a descent of which we become not only spiritually but physically conscious. The siddhi or full accomplishment of this movement can only come when we are able to lift the centre of thought and conscious action above the physical brain and feel it going on in the subtle body. If we can feel ourselves thinking no longer with the brain but from above and outside the head in the subtle body, that is a sure physical sign of a release from the limitations of the physical mind, and though this will not be complete at once nor of itself bring the supramental action, for the subtle body is mental and not supramental, still it is a subtle and pure mentality and makes an easier communication with the supramental centres. The lower movements must still come, but it is then found easier to arrive at a swift and subtle discrimination telling us at once the difference, distinguishing the intuitional thought from the lower intellectual mixture, separating it from its mental coatings, rejecting the mere rapidities of the mind which imitate the form of the intuition without being of its true substance. It will be easier to discern rapidly the higher planes of the true supramental being and call down their power to effect the desired transformation and to refer all the lower action to the superior power and light that it may reject and eliminate, purify and transform and select among them its right material for the Truth that has to be organised within us. This opening up of a higher level and of higher and higher planes of it and the consequent re-formation of our whole consciousness and its action into their mould and into the substance of their power and luminous capacity is found in practice to be the greater part of the natural method used by the divine Shakti.

A fourth method is one which suggests itself naturally to the developed intelligence and suits the thinking man. This is to develop our intellect instead of eliminating it, but with the will not to cherish its limitations, but to heighten its capacity, light, intensity, degree and force of activity until it borders on the thing that transcends it and can easily be taken up and transformed into that higher conscious action. This movement also is founded on the truth of our nature and enters into the course and movement of the complete Yoga of self-perfection. That course, as I have described it, included a heightening and greatening of the action of our natural instruments and powers till they constitute in their purity and essential completeness a preparatory perfection of the present normal movement of the Shakti that acts in us. The reason and intelligent will, the buddhi, is the greatest of these powers and instruments, the natural leader of the rest in the developed human being, the most capable of aiding the development of the others. The ordinary activities of our nature are all of them of use for the greater perfection we seek, are meant to be turned into material for them, and the greater their development, the richer the preparation for the supramental action.

The intellectual being too has to be taken up by the Shakti in the Yoga and raised to its fullest and its most heightened powers. The subsequent transformation of the intellect is possible because all the action of the intellect derives secretly from the supermind, each thought and will contains some truth of it however limited and altered by the inferior action of the intelligence. The transformation can be brought about by the removal of the limitation and the elimination of the distorting or perverting element. This however cannot be done by the heightening and greatening of the intellectual activity alone; for that must always be limited by the original inherent defects of the mental intelligence. An intervention of the supramental energy is needed that can light up and get rid of its deficiencies of thought and will and feeling. This intervention too cannot be completely effective unless the supramental plane is manifested and acts above the mind no longer from behind a lid or veil, however thin the veil may have grown, but more constantly in an open and luminous action till there is seen the full sun of Truth with no cloud to moderate its splendour. It is not necessary, either, to develop the intellect fully in its separateness before calling down this intervention or opening up by it the supramental levels. The intervention may come in earlier and at once develop the intellectual action and turn it, as it develops, into the higher intuitive form and substance.

The widest natural action of the Shakti combines all these methods. It creates, sometimes at first, sometimes at some later, perhaps latest stage, the freedom of the spiritual silence. It opens the secret intuitive being within the mind itself and accustoms us to refer all our thought and our feeling and will and action to the initiation of the Divine, the Splendour and Power who is now concealed in the heart of its recesses. It raises, when we are ready, the centre of its operations to the mental summit and opens up the supramental levels and proceeds doubly by an action from above downward filling and transforming the lower nature and an action from below upwards raising all the energies to that which is above them till the transcendence is completed and the change of the whole system integrally effected. It takes and develops the intelligence and will and other natural powers, but brings in constantly the intuitive mind and afterwards the true supramental energy to change and enlarge their action. These things it does in no fixed and mechanically invariable order, such as the rigidity of the logical intellect might demand, but freely and flexibly according to the needs of its work and the demand of the nature.

The first result will not be the creation of the true supermind, but the organisation of a predominantly or even a completely intuitive mentality sufficiently developed to take the place of the ordinary mentality and of the logical reasoning intellect of the developed human being. The most prominent change will be the transmutation of the thought heightened and filled by that substance of concentrated light, concentrated power, concentrated joy of the light and the power and that direct accuracy which are the marks of a true intuitive thinking. It is not only primary suggestions or rapid conclusions that this mind will give, but it will conduct too with the same light, power, joy of sureness and direct spontaneous seeing of the truth the connecting and developing operations now conducted by the intellectual reason. The will also will be changed into this intuitive character, proceed directly with light and power to the thing to be done, *kartavyaṁ karma*, and dispose with a rapid sight of possibilities and actualities the combinations necessary to its action and its purpose. The feelings also will be intuitive, seizing upon right relations, acting with a new light and power and a glad sureness, retaining only right and spontaneous desires and emotions, so long as these things endure, and, when they pass away, replacing them by a luminous and spontaneous love and an Ananda that knows and seizes at once on the right *rasa* of its objects. All the other mental movements will be similarly enlightened and even too the pranic and sense movements and the consciousness of the body. And usually there will be some development also of the psychic faculties, powers and perceptions of the inner mind and its senses not dependent on the outer sense and the reason. The intuitive mentality will be not only a stronger and a more luminous thing, but usually capable of a much more extensive operation than the ordinary mind of the same man before this development of the Yoga.

This intuitive mentality, if it could be made perfect in its nature, unmixed with any inferior element and yet unconscious of its own limitations and of the greatness of the thing beyond it, might form another definite status and halting place like the instinctive mind of the animal or the reasoning mind of man. But the intuitive mentality cannot be made abidingly perfect and self-sufficient except by the opening power of the supermind above it and that at once reveals its limitations and makes of it a secondary action transitional between the intellectual mind and the true supramental nature. The intuitive mentality is still mind and not gnosis. It is indeed a light from the supermind, but modified and diminished by the stuff of mind in which it works, and stuff of mind means always a basis of ignorance. The intuitive mind is not yet the wide sunlight of truth, but a constant play of flashes of it keeping lighted up a basic state of ignorance or of half-knowledge and indirect knowledge. As long as it is imperfect, it is invaded by a mixture of ignorant mentality which crosses its truth with a strain of error. After it has acquired a larger native action more free from this intermixture, even then so long as the stuff of mind in which it works is capable of the old intellectual or lower mental habit, it is subject to accretion of error, to clouding, to many kinds of relapse. Moreover the individual mind does not live alone and to itself but in the general mind and all that it has rejected is discharged into the general mind atmosphere around it and tends to return upon and invade it with the old suggestions and many promptings of the old mental character. The intuitive mind, growing or grown, has therefore to be constantly on guard against invasion and accretion, on the watch to reject and eliminate immixtures, busy intuitivising more and still more the whole stuff of mind, and this can only end by itself being enlightened, transformed, lifted up into the full light of the supramental being.

Moreover, this new mentality is in each man a development of the present power of his being and, however new and remarkable its developments, its organisation is within a certain range of capacity. Adventuring beyond that border—it may indeed limit itself to the work in hand and its present range of realised capacity, but the nature of a mind opened to the infinite is to progress and change and enlarge—it there becomes liable to a return, however modified by the new intuitive habit, of the old intellectual seeking in the ignorance,—unless and until it is constantly overtopped and led by the manifested action of a fuller supramental luminous energy. This is indeed its nature that it is a link and transition between present mind and the supermind and, so long as the transition is not complete, there is sometimes a gravitation downward, sometimes a tendency upward, an oscillation, an invasion and attraction from below, an invasion and attraction from above, and at best an uncertain and limited status between the two poles. As the higher intelligence of man is situated between his animal and customary human mind below and his evolving spiritual mind above, so this first spiritual mind is situated between the intellectualised human mentality and the greater supramental knowledge.

The nature of mind is that it lives between half-lights and darkness, amid probabilities and possibilities, amid partly grasped aspects, amid incertitudes and half certitudes: it is an ignorance grasping at knowledge, striving to enlarge itself and pressing against the concealed body of true gnosis. The supermind lives in the light of spiritual certitudes: it is to man knowledge opening the actual body of its own native effulgence. The intuitive mind appears at first a lightening up of the mind's half-lights, its probabilities and possibilities, its aspects, its uncertain certitudes, its representations, and a revealing of the truth concealed or half concealed and half manifested by these things, and in its higher action it is a first bringing of the supramental truth by a nearer directness of seeing, a luminous indication or memory of the spirit's knowledge, an intuition or looking in through the gates of the being's secret universal self-vision and knowledge. It is a first imperfect organisation of that greater light and power, imperfect because done in the mind, not based on its own native substance of consciousness, a constant communication, but not a quite immediate and constant presence. The perfect perfection lies beyond on the supramental levels and must be based on a more decisive and complete transformation of the mentality and of our whole nature.

# THE GRADATIONS OF THE SUPERMIND

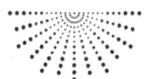

THE INTUITIVE MIND is an immediate translation of truth into mental terms half transformed by a radiant supramental substance, a translation of some infinite self-knowledge that acts above mind in the superconscient spirit. That spirit becomes conscient to us as a greater self at once above and in and around us of which our present self, our mental, vital and physical personality and nature, is an imperfect portion or a partial derivation or an inferior and inadequate symbol, and as the intuitive mind grows in us, as our whole being grows more moulded to an intuitive substance, we feel a sort of half transformation of our members into the nature of this greater self and spirit. All our thought, will, impulse, feeling, even in the end our more outward vital and physical sensations become more and more direct transmissions from the spirit and are of another and a more and more pure, untroubled, powerful and luminous nature. This is one side of the change: the other is that whatever belongs still to the lower being, whatever still seems to us to come from outside or as a survival of the action of our old inferior personality, feels the pressure of the change and increasingly tends to modify and transform itself to the new substance and nature. The higher comes down and largely takes the place of the lower, but also the lower changes, transforms itself into material of the action and becomes part of the substance of the higher being.

The greater spirit above the mind appears at first as a presence, a light, a power, a source, an infinite, but all that is knowable to us in it is at first an infinite identity of being, consciousness, power of consciousness, Ananda. The rest comes from it, but takes no determinate shape of thought, will or feeling above us, but only in the intuitive mind and on its level. Or we feel and are manifoldly aware of a great and infinite Purusha who is the eternally living truth of that being and presence, a great and infinite knowledge which is the potency of that light and consciousness, a great and infinite will which is the potency of that power of consciousness, a great and infinite love which is the potency of that Ananda. But all these potencies are only known to us in any definite manner, apart from the strong reality and effect of their essential presence, in so far as they are translated to our intuitive mental being and on its level and within its limits. As however we progress or as we grow into a more luminous and dynamic union with that spirit or Purusha, a greater action of knowledge and will and spiritual feeling manifests and seems to organise itself above the mind and this we recognise as the true supermind and the real native play of the infinite knowledge, will and Ananda. The intuitive mentality then becomes a secondary and inferior movement waiting upon this higher power, responding and assenting to all its illuminations and dictates, transmitting them to the lower members, and, when they do not arrive or are not in immediate evidence, often attempting to supply its place, imitate its action and do as best it can the works of the supramental nature. It takes in fact the same place and relation with regard to it as was taken with regard to itself by the ordinary intelligence at an earlier stage of the Yoga.

This double action on the two planes of our being at first strengthens the intuitive mentality as a secondary operation and assists it to expel or transform more completely the survivals or invasions or accretions of the ignorance. And more and more it intensifies the intuitive mentality itself in its light of knowledge and eventually transforms it into the image of the supermind itself, but at first, ordinarily, in the more limited action of the gnosis when it takes the form of what we might call a luminous supramental or divine reason. It is as this divine reason that the supermind itself at the beginning may manifest its action and then, when it has changed the mind into its own image, it descends and takes the place of the ordinary intelligence and reason. Meanwhile a higher supramental power of a much greater character has been revealing itself above which takes the supreme lead of the divine action in the being. The divine reason is of a more limited character because, although not of the mental stamp and although an operation of the direct truth and knowledge, it is a delegated power for a range of purposes greater in light, but still to a certain extent analogous to those of the ordinary human will and reason; it is in the yet greater supermind that there comes the direct, altogether revealed and immediate action of the Ishwara in the human being. These distinctions between the intuitive mind, the divine reason and the greater supermind, and others within these gradations themselves, have to be made because eventually they become of great importance. At first the mind takes all that comes from beyond it without distinction as the sufficient spiritual illumination and accepts even initial states and first enlightenments as a finality, but afterwards it finds that to rest here would be to rest in a partial realisation and that one has to go on heightening and enlarging till at least there is reached a certain completeness of divine breadth and stature.

It is difficult for the intellect to grasp at all what is meant by these supramental distinctions: the mental terms in which they can be rendered are lacking or inadequate and they can only be understood after a certain sight or certain approximations in experience. A number of indications are all that at present it can be useful to give. And first it will be enough to take certain clues from the thinking mind; for it is there that some of the nearest keys to the supramental action are discoverable. The thought of the intuitive mind proceeds wholly by four powers that shape the form of the truth, an intuition that suggests its idea, an intuition that discriminates, an inspiration that brings in its word and something of its greater substance and a revelation that shapes to the sight its very face and body of reality. These things are not the same as certain movements of the ordinary mental intelligence that look analogous and are easily mistaken for the true intuition in our first inexperience. The suggestive intuition is not the same thing as the intellectual insight of a quick intelligence or the intuitive discrimination as the rapid judgment of the reasoning intellect; the intuitive inspiration is not the same as the inspired action of the imaginative intelligence, nor the intuitive revelation as the strong light of a purely mental close seizing and experience.

It would perhaps be accurate to say that these latter activities are mental representations of the higher movements, attempts of the ordinary mind to do the same things or the best possible imitations the intellect can offer of the functionings of the higher nature. The true intuitions differ from these effective but insufficient counterfeits in their substance of light, their operation, their method of knowledge. The intellectual rapidities are dependent on awakenings of the basic mental ignorance to mental figures and representations of truth that may be quite valid in their own field and for their own purpose but are not necessarily and by their very nature reliable. They are dependent for their emergence on the suggestions given by mental and sense data or on the accumulation of past mental knowledge. They search for the truth as a thing outside, an object to be found and looked at and stored as an acquisition and, when found, scrutinise its surfaces, suggestions or aspects. This scrutiny can never give a quite complete and adequate truth idea. However positive they may seem at the time, they may at any moment have to be passed over, rejected and found inconsistent with fresh knowledge.

The intuitive knowledge on the contrary, however limited it may be in its field or application, is within that scope sure with an immediate, a durable and especially a self-existent certitude. It may take for starting-point or rather for a thing to light up and disclose in its true sense the data of mind and sense or else fire a train of past thought and knowledge to new meanings and issues, but it is dependent on nothing but itself and may leap out of its own field of lustres, independent of previous suggestion or data, and this kind of action becomes progressively more common and adds itself to the other to initiate new depths and ranges of knowledge. In either case there is always an element of self-existent truth and a sense of absoluteness of origination suggestive of its proceeding from the spirit's knowledge by identity. It is the disclosing of a knowledge that is secret but already existent in the being: it is not an acquisition, but something that was always there and revealable. It sees the truth from within and illumines with that inner vision the outsides and it harmonises, too, readily—provided we keep intuitively awake—with whatever fresh truth has yet to arrive. These characteristics become more pronounced and intense in the higher, the proper supramental ranges: in the intuitive mind they may not be always recognisable in their purity and completeness, because of the mixture of mental stuff and its accretion, but in the divine reason and greater supramental action they become free and absolute.

The suggestive intuition acting on the mental level suggests a direct and illumining inner idea of the truth, an idea that is its true image and index, not as yet the entirely present and whole sight, but rather of the nature of a bright memory of some truth, a recognition of a secret of the self's knowledge. It is a representation, but a living representation, not an ideative symbol, a reflection, but a reflection that is lit up with something of the truth's real substance. The intuitive discrimination is a secondary action setting this idea of the truth in its right place and its relation to other ideas. And so long as there is the habit of mental interference and accretion it works also to separate the mental from the higher seeing, to discrete the inferior mental stuff that embarrasses with its alloy the pure truth substance, and labours to unravel the mingled skein of ignorance and knowledge, falsehood and error. As the intuition is of the nature of a memory, a luminous remembering of the self-existent truth, so the inspiration is of the nature of truth hearing: it is an immediate reception of the very voice of the truth, it readily brings the word that perfectly embodies it and it carries something more than the light of its idea; there is seized some stream of its inner reality and vivid arriving movement of its substance. The revelation is of the nature of direct sight, *pratyakṣa-dṛṣṭi*, and makes evident to a present vision the thing in itself of which the idea is the representation. It brings out the very spirit and being and reality of the truth and makes it part of the consciousness and the experience.

In the actual process of the development of the supramental nature, supposing it to follow a regular gradation, it may be seen that the two lower powers come out first, though not necessarily void of all action of the two higher powers, and as they increase and become a normal action, they make a sort of lower intuitive gnosis. The combination of the two together is necessary for its completeness. If the intuitive discrimination works by itself, it creates a sort of critical illumination that acts on the ideas and perceptions of the intellect and turns them on themselves in such a way that the mind can separate their truth from their error. It creates in the end in place of the intellectual judgment a luminous intuitive judgment, a sort of critical gnosis: but it is likely to be deficient in fresh illuminative knowledge or to create only so much extension of truth as is the natural consequence of the separation of error. On the other hand, if the suggestive intuition works by itself without this discrimination, there is indeed a constant accession of new truths and new lights, but they are easily surrounded and embarrassed by the mental accretions and their connections and relation or harmonious development out of each other are clouded and broken by the interference. A normalised power of active intuitive perception is created, but not any complete and coherent mind of intuitive gnosis. The two together supply the deficiencies of each other's single action and build up a mind of intuitive perception and discrimination which can do the work and more than the work of the stumbling mental intelligence and do it with the greater light, surety and power of a more direct and unfaltering ideation.

The two higher powers in the same way make a higher intuitive gnosis. Acting as separate powers in the mentality they too are not in themselves sufficient without the companion activities. The revelation may indeed present the reality, the identities of the thing in itself and add something of great power to the experience of the conscious being, but it may lack the embodying word, the out-bringing idea, the connected pursuit of its relations and consequences and may remain a possession in the self but not a thing communicated to and through the members. There may be the presence of the truth but not its full manifestation. The inspiration may give the word of the truth and the stir of its dynamis and movement, but this is not a complete thing and sure in its effect without the full revelation of all that it bears in itself and luminously indicates and the ordering of it in its relations. The inspired intuitive mind is a mind of lightnings lighting up many things that were dark, but the light needs to be canalised and fixed into a stream of steady lustres that will be a constant power for lucidly ordered knowledge. The higher gnosis by itself in its two sole powers would be a mind of spiritual splendours living too much in its own separate domain, producing perhaps invisibly its effect on the outside world, but lacking the link of a more close and ordinary communication with its more normal movements that is provided by the lower ideative action. It is the united or else the fused and unified action of the four powers that makes the complete and fully armed and equipped intuitive gnosis.

A regular development would at first, allowing for some simultaneous manifestation of the four powers, yet create on a sufficiently extensive scale the lower suggestive and critical intuitive mind and then develop above it the inspired and the revelatory intuitive mentality. Next it would take up the two lower powers into the power and field of the inspiration and make all act as one harmony doing simultaneously the united—or, at a higher intensity, indistinguishably as one light the unified—action of the three. And last it would execute a similar movement of taking up into and fusion with the revelatory power of the intuitive gnosis. As a matter of fact in the human mind the clear process of the development is likely always to be more or less disturbed, confused and rendered irregular in its course, subjected to relapses, incomplete advances, returns upon things unaccomplished or imperfectly accomplished owing to the constant mixture and intervention of the existing movements of the mental half-knowledge and the obstruction of the stuff of the mental ignorance. In the end however a time can come when the process, so far as it is possible in the mind itself, is complete and a clear formation of a modified supramental light is possible composed of all these powers, the highest leading or absorbing into its own body the others. It is at this point, when the intuitive mind has been fully formed in the mental being and is strong enough to dominate if not yet wholly to occupy the various mental activities, that a farther step becomes possible, the lifting of the centre and level of action above the mind and the predominance of the supramental reason.

The first character of this change is a complete reversal, a turning over, one might almost say, upside down of the whole activity. At present we live in the mind and mostly in the physical mind, but still not entirely involved like the animal in the physical, vital and sensational workings. On the contrary we have attained to a certain mental elevation from which we can look down on the action of the life, sense and body, turn the higher mental light on them, reflect, judge, use our will to modify the action of the inferior nature. On the other hand we look up too from that elevation more or less consciously to something above and receive from it either directly or through our subconscient or subliminal being some secret superconscient impulsion of our thought and will and other activities. The process of this communication is veiled and obscure and men are not ordinarily aware of it except in certain highly developed natures: but when we advance in self-knowledge, we find that all our thought and will originate from above though formed in the mind and there first overtly active. If we release the knots of the physical mind which binds us to the brain instrument and identifies us with the bodily consciousness and can move in the pure mentality, this becomes constantly clear to the perception.

The development of the intuitive mentality makes this communication direct, no longer subconscient and obscure; but we are still in the mind and the mind still looks upward and receives the supramental communication and passes it on to the other members. In doing so it no longer wholly creates its own form for the thought and will that come down to it, but still it modifies and qualifies and limits them and imposes something of its own method. It is still the receiver and the transmitter of the thought and will,—though not formative of them now except by a subtle influence, because it provides them or at least surrounds them with a mental stuff or a mental setting and framework and atmosphere. When however the supramental reason develops, the Purusha rises above the mental elevation and now looks down on the whole action of mind, life, sense, body from quite another light and atmosphere, sees and knows it with quite a different vision and, because he is no longer involved in the mind, with a free and true knowledge. Man is at present only partly liberated from the animal involution,—for his mind is partially lifted above, partially immerged and controlled by the life, sense and body,—and he is not at all liberated from the mental forms and limits. But after he rises to the supramental elevation, he is delivered from the nether control and governor of his whole nature—essentially and initially only at first and in his highest consciousness, for the rest remains still to be transformed,—but when or in proportion as that is done, he becomes a free being and master of his mind, sense, life and body.

The second character of the change is that the formation of the thought and will can take place now wholly on the supramental level and therefore there is initiated an entirely luminous and effective will and knowledge. The light and the power are not indeed complete at the beginning because the supramental reason is only an elementary formulation of the supermind and because the mind and other members have yet to be changed into the mould of the supramental nature. The mind, it is true, no longer acts as the apparent originator, formulator or judge of the thought and will or anything else, but it still acts as the transmitting channel and therefore in that degree as a recipient and to a certain extent an obstructor and qualifier in transmission of the power and light that comes from above. There is a disparateness between the supramental consciousness in which the Purusha now stands, thinks and wills and the mental, vital and physical consciousness through which he has to effectuate its light and knowledge. He lives and sees with an ideal consciousness, but he has yet in his lower self to make it entirely practical and effective. Otherwise he can only act with a greater or less spiritual effectiveness through an internal communication with others on the spiritual level and on the higher mental level that is most easily affected by it, but the effect is diminished and is retarded by the inferiority or lack of the integral play of the being. This can only be remedied by the supermind taking hold of and supramentalising the mental, the vital and the physical consciousness,—transforming them, that is to say, into moulds of the supramental nature. This is much more easily done if there has been that Yogic preparation of the instruments of the lower nature of which I have already spoken; otherwise there is much difficulty in getting rid of the discord or disparateness between the ideal supramentality and the mental transmitting instruments, the mind channel, the heart, the sense, the nervous and the physical being. The supramental reason can do the first and a fairly ample, though not the entire work of this transformation.

The supramental reason is of the nature of a spiritual, direct, self-luminous, self-acting will and intelligence not mental, *mānasa buddhi*, but supramental, *vijñāna buddhi*. It acts by the same four powers as the intuitive mind, but these powers are here active in an initial fullness of body not modified by the mental stuff of the intelligence, not concerned mainly with an illumining of the mind, but at work in their own proper manner and for their own native purpose. And of these four the discrimination here is hardly recognisable as a separate power, but is constantly inherent in the three others and is their own determination of the scope and relations of their knowledge. There are three elevations in this reason, one in which the action of what we may call a supramental intuition gives the form and the predominant character, one in which a rapid supramental inspiration and one in which a large supramental revelation leads and imparts the general character, and each of these raises us to a more concentrated substance and a higher light, sufficiency and scope of the truth will and the truth knowledge.

The work of the supramental reason covers and goes beyond all that is done by the mental reason, but it starts from the other end and has a corresponding operation. The essential truths of self and the spirit and the principle of things are not to the spiritual reason abstract ideas or subtle unsubstantial experiences to which it arrives by a sort of overleaping of limits, but a constant reality and the natural background of all its ideation and experience. It does not like the mind arrive at, but discloses directly both the general and total and the particular truths of being and consciousness, of spiritual and other sensation and Ananda and of force and action,—reality and phenomenon and symbol, actuality and possibility and eventuality, that which is determined and that which determines, and all with a self-luminous evidence. It formulates and arranges the relations of thought and thought, of force and force, of action and action and of all these with each other and throws them into a convincing and luminous harmony. It includes the data of sense, but gives to them another meaning in the light of what is behind them, and treats them only as outermost indications: the inner truth is known to a greater sense which it already possesses. And it is not dependent on them alone even in their own field of objects or limited by their range. It has a spiritual sense and sensation of its own and it takes and relates to that the data too of a sixth sense, the inner mind sense. And it takes also the illuminations and the living symbols and images familiar to the psychic experience and relates these too to the truths of the self and spirit.

The spiritual reason takes also the emotions and psychic sensations, relates them to their spiritual equivalents and imparts to them the values of the higher consciousness and Ananda from which they derive and are its modifications in an inferior nature and it corrects their deformations. It takes similarly the movements of the vital being and consciousness and relates them to the movements and imparts to them the significances of the spiritual life of the self and its power of Tapas. It takes the physical consciousness, delivers it from its darkness and tamas of inertia and makes it a responsive recipient and a sensitive instrument of the supramental light and power and Ananda. It deals with life and action and knowledge like the mental will and reason, but not starting from matter, life and sense and their data and relating to them through the idea the truth of higher things, but it starts on the contrary from truth of self and spirit and relates to that through a direct spiritual experience assuming all other experience as its forms and instruments the things of mind and soul and life and sense and matter. It commands a far vaster range than the ordinary embodied mind shut up in the prison of the physical senses and vaster too than the pure mentality, even when that is free in its own ranges and operates with the aid of the psychical mind and inner senses. And it has that power which the mental will and reason do not possess, because they are not truly self-determined and originally determinative of things, the power of transforming the whole being in all its parts into a harmonious instrument and manifestation of the spirit.

At the same time the spiritual reason acts mainly by the representative idea and will in the spirit, though it has a greater and more essential truth as its constant source and supporter and reference. It is, then, a power of light of the Ishwara, but not the very self-power of his immediate presence in the being; it is his *sūrya-śakti*, not his whole *ātma-śakti* or *parā svā prakṛti*, that works in the spiritual reason. The immediate self-power begins its direct operation in the greater supermind, and that takes up all that has hitherto been realised in body, life and mind and in the intuitive being and by the spiritual reason and shapes all that has been created, all that has been gathered, turned into stuff of experience and made part of the consciousness, personality and nature by the mental being, into a highest harmony with the high infinite and universal life of the spirit. The mind can have the touch of the infinite and the universal and can reflect and even lose itself in them, but the supermind alone can enable the individual to be completely one in action with the universal and transcendent spirit.

Here the one thing that is always and constantly present, that which one has grown to and in which one lives always, is infinite being and all that is is seen, felt, known, existed in as only substance of the one being; it is infinite consciousness and all that is conscious and acts and moves is seen, felt, received, known, lived in as self-experience and energy of the one being; it is infinite Ananda and all that feels and is felt is seen and felt and known, received and lived in as forms of the one Ananda. Everything else is only manifestation and circumstance of this one truth of our existence. This is no longer merely the seeing or knowing, but the very condition of the self in all and all in the self, God in all and all in God and all seen as God, and that condition is now not a thing offered to the reflecting spiritualised mind but held and lived by an integral, always present, always active realisation in the supramental nature. There is thought here and will and sensation and everything that belongs to our nature, but it is transfigured and elevated into a higher consciousness. All thought is here seen and experienced as a luminous body of substance, a luminous movement of force, a luminous wave of Ananda of the being; it is not an idea in the void air of mind, but experienced in the reality and as the light of a reality of the infinite being. The will and impulsions are similarly experienced as a real power and substance of the Sat, the Chit, the Ananda of the Ishwara. All the spiritualised sensation and emotion are experienced as pure moulds of the consciousness and Ananda. The physical being itself is experienced as a conscious form and the vital being as an outpouring of the power and possession of the life of the spirit.

The action of the supermind in the development is to manifest and organise this highest consciousness so as to exist and act no longer only in the infinite above with some limited or veiled or lower and deformed manifestations in the individual being and nature, but largely and totally in the individual as a conscious and self-knowing spiritual being and a living and acting power of the infinite and universal spirit. The character of this action, so far as it can be expressed, may be spoken of more fitly afterwards when we come to speak of the Brahmic consciousness and vision. In the succeeding chapters we shall only deal with so much of it as concerns the thought, will and psychic and other experience in the individual nature. At present all that is necessary to note is that here too there is in the field of the thought and the will a triple action. The spiritual reason is lifted and broadened into a greater representative action that formulates to us mainly the actualities of the existence of the self in and around us. There is then a higher interpretative action of the supramental knowledge, a greater scale less insistent on actualities, that opens out yet greater potentialities in time and space and beyond. And lastly there is a highest knowledge by identity that is a gate of entrance to the essential self-awareness and the omniscience and omnipotence of the Ishwara.

It must not however be supposed that these superimposed stages are shut off in experience from each other. I have placed them in what might be a regular order of ascending development for the better possibility of understanding in an intellectual statement. But the infinite even in the normal mind breaks through its own veils and across its own dividing lines of descent and ascension and gives often intimations of itself in one manner or another. And while we are still in the intuitive mentality, the things above open and come to us in irregular visitations, then form as we grow a more frequent and regularised action above it. These anticipations are still more large and frequent the moment we enter on the supramental level. The universal and infinite consciousness can always seize on and surround the mind and it is when it does so with a certain continuity, frequency or persistence that the mind can most easily transform itself into the intuitive mentality and that again into the supramental movement. Only as we rise we grow more intimately and integrally into the infinite consciousness and it becomes more fully our own self and nature. And also, on the other, the lower side of existence which it might seem would then be not only beneath but quite alien to us, even when we live in the supramental being and even when the whole nature has been formed into its mould, that need not cut us off from the knowledge and feeling of others who live in the ordinary nature. The lower or more limited may have a difficulty in understanding and feeling the higher, but the higher and less limited can always, if it will, understand and identify itself with the lower nature. The supreme Ishwara too is not aloof from us; he knows, lives in, identifies himself with all and yet is not subjugated by the reactions or limited in his knowledge, power and Ananda by the limitations of the mind and life and physical being in the universe.

# THE SUPRAMENTAL THOUGHT AND KNOWLEDGE

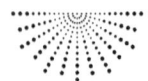

THE TRANSITION from mind to supermind is not only the substitution of a greater instrument of thought and knowledge, but a change and conversion of the whole consciousness. There is evolved not only a supramental thought, but a supramental will, sense, feeling, a supramental substitute for all the activities that are now accomplished by the mind. All these higher activities are first manifested in the mind itself as descents, irruptions, messages or revelations of a superior power. Mostly they are mixed up with the more ordinary action of the mind and not easily distinguishable from them in our first inexperience except by their superior light and force and joy, the more so as the mind greatened or excited by their frequent coming quickens its own action and imitates the external characteristics of the supramental activity: its own operation is made more swift, luminous, strong and positive and it arrives even at a kind of imitative and often false intuition that strives to be but is not really the luminous, direct and self-existent truth. The next step is the formation of a luminous mind of intuitive experience, thought, will, feeling, sense from which the intermixture of the lesser mind and the imitative intuition are progressively eliminated: this is a process of purification, *śuddhi*, necessary to the new formation and perfection, *siddhi*. At the same time there is the disclosure above the mind of the source of the intuitive action and a more and more organised functioning of a true supramental consciousness acting not in the mind but on its own higher plane. This draws up into itself in the end the intuitive mentality it has created as its representative and assumes the charge of the whole activity of the consciousness. The process is progressive and for a long time chequered by admixture and the necessity of a return upon the lower movements in order to correct and transform them. The higher and the lower power act sometimes alternately,—the consciousness descending back from the heights it had attained to its former level but always with some change,—but sometimes together and with a sort of mutual reference. The mind eventually becomes wholly intuitivised and exists only as a passive channel for the supramental action; but this condition too is not ideal and presents, besides, still a certain obstacle, because the higher action has still to pass through a retarding and diminishing conscious substance,—that of the physical consciousness. The final stage of the change will come when the supermind occupies and supramentalises the whole being and turns even the vital and physical sheaths into mould of itself, responsive, subtle and instinct with its powers. Man then becomes wholly the superman. This is at least the natural and integral process.

It would be to go altogether outside present limits to attempt anything like an adequate presentation of the whole character of the supermind; and it would not be possible to give a complete presentation, since the supermind carries in it the unity, but also the largeness and multiplicities of the infinite. All that need now be done is to present some salient characters from the point of view of the actual process of the conversion in the Yoga, the relation to the action of mind and the principle of some of the phenomena of the change. This is the fundamental relation that all the action of the mind is a derivation from the secret supermind, although we do not know this until we come to know our higher self, and draws from that source all it has of truth and value. All our thoughts, willings, feelings, sense representations have in them or at their roots an element of truth, which originates and sustains their existence, however in the actuality they may be perverted or false, and behind them a greater ungrasped truth, which if they could grasp it, would make them soon unified, harmonious and at least relatively complete. Actually, however, such truth as they have is diminished in scope, degraded into a lower movement, divided and falsified by fragmentation, afflicted with incompleteness, marred by perversion. Mental knowledge is not an integral but always a partial knowledge. It adds constantly detail to detail, but has a difficulty in relating them aright; its wholes too are not real but incomplete wholes which it tends to substitute for the more real and integral knowledge. And even if it arrived at a kind of integral knowledge, it would still be by a sort of putting together, a mental and intellectual arrangement, an artificial unity and not an essential and real oneness. If that were all, the mind might conceivably arrive at some kind of half reflection half translation of an integral knowledge, but the radical malady would still be that it would not be the real thing, but only at best an intellectual representation. That the mental truth must always be, an intellectual, emotional and sensational representation, not the direct truth, not truth itself in its body and essence.

The supermind can do all that the mind does, present and combine details and what might be called aspects or subordinate wholes, but it does it in a different way and on another basis. It does not like the mind bring in the element of deviation, false extension and imposed error, but even when it gives a partial knowledge, gives it in a firm and exact light, and always there is behind implied or opened to the consciousness the essential truth on which the details and subordinate wholes or aspects depend. The supermind has also a power of representation, but its representations are not of the intellectual kind, they are filled with the body and substance of light of the truth in its essence, they are its vehicles and not substituted figures. There is such an infinite power of representation of the supermind and that is the divine power of which the mental action is a sort of fallen representative. This representative supermind has a lower action in what I have called the supramental reason, nearest to the mental and into which the mental can most easily be taken up, and a higher action in the integral supermind that sees all things in the unity and infinity of the divine consciousness and self-existence. But on whatever level, it is a different thing from the corresponding mental action, direct, luminous, secure. The whole inferiority of the mind comes from its being the action of the soul after it has fallen into the nescience and the ignorance and is trying to get back to self-knowledge but doing it still on the basis of the nescience and the ignorance. The mind is the ignorance attempting to know or it is the ignorance receiving a derivative knowledge: it is the action of Avidya. The supermind is always the disclosure of an inherent and self-existent knowledge; it is the action of Vidya.

A second difference that we experience is a greater and a spontaneous harmony and unity. All consciousness is one, but in action it takes on many movements and each of these fundamental movements has many forms and processes. The forms and processes of the mind consciousness are marked by a disturbing and perplexing division and separateness of the mental energies and movements in which the original unity of the conscious mind does not at all or only distractedly appears. Constantly we find in our mentality a conflict or else a confusion and want of combination between different thoughts or a patched up combination and the same phenomenon applies to the various movements of our will and desire and to our emotions and feelings. Again our thought and our will and our feeling are not in a state of natural harmony and unison with each other, but act in their separate power even when they have to act together and are frequently in conflict or to some degree at variance. There is too an unequal development of one at the expense of another. The mind is a thing of discords in which some kind of practical arrangement rather than a satisfying concord is established for the purposes of life. The reason tries to arrive at a better arrangement, aims at a better control, a rational or an ideal harmony, and in this attempt it is a delegate or substitute of the supermind and is trying to do what only the supermind can do in its own right: but actually it is not able wholly to control the rest of the being and there is usually a considerable difference between the rational or ideal harmony we create in our thoughts and the movement of the life. Even at the best the arrangement made by the reason has always in it something of artificiality and imposition, for in the end there are only two spontaneous harmonic movements, that of the life, inconscient or largely subconscient, the harmony that we find in the animal creation and in lower Nature, and that of the spirit. The human condition is a stage of transition, effort and imperfection between the one and the other, between the natural and the ideal or spiritual life and it is full of uncertain seeking and disorder. It is not that the mental being cannot find or rather construct some kind of relative harmony of its own, but that it cannot render it stable because it is under the urge of the spirit. Man is obliged by a Power within him to be the labourer of a more or less conscious self-evolution that shall lead him to self-mastery and self-knowledge.

The supermind in its action is on the contrary a thing of unity and harmony and inherent order. At first when the pressure from above falls on the mentality, this is not realised and even a contrary phenomenon may for a time appear. That is due to several causes. First, there may be a disturbance, even a derangement created by impact of the greater hardly measurable power on an inferior consciousness which is not capable of responding to it organically or even perhaps of bearing the pressure. The very fact of the simultaneous and yet uncoordinated activity of two quite different forces, especially if the mind insists on its own way, if it tries obstinately or violently to profit by the supermind instead of giving itself up to it and its purpose, if it is not sufficiently passive and obedient to the higher guidance, may lead to a great excitation of power but also an increased disorder. It is for this reason that a previous preparation and long purification, the more complete the better, and a tranquillising and ordinarily a passivity of the mind calmly and strongly open to the spirit are necessities of the Yoga.

Again the mind, accustomed to act in limits, may try to supramentalise itself on the line of any one of its energies. It may develop a considerable power of intuitive half-supramentalised thought and knowledge, but the will may remain untransformed and out of harmony with this partial half-supramental development of the thinking mind, and the rest of the being too, emotional and nervous, may continue to be equally or more unregenerate. Or there may be a very great development of intuitive or strongly inspired will, but no corresponding uplifting of the thought mind or the emotional and psychic being, or only at most so much as is specially needed in order not wholly to obstruct the will action. The emotional or psychic mind may try to intuitivise and supramentalise itself and to a great extent succeed, and yet the thinking mind remain ordinary, poor in stuff and obscure in its light. There may be a development of intuitivity in the ethical or aesthetic being, but the rest may remain very much as it was. This is the reason of the frequent disorder or one-sidedness which we mark in the man of genius, poet, artist, thinker, saint or mystic. A partially intuitivised mentality may present an appearance of much less harmony and order outside its special activity than the largely developed intellectual mind. An integral development is needed, a wholesale conversion of the mind; otherwise the action is that of the mind using the supramental influx for its own profit and in its own mould, and that is allowed for the immediate purpose of the Divine in the being and may even be considered as a stage sufficient for the individual in this one life: but it is a state of imperfection and not the complete and successful evolution of the being. If however there is an integral development of the intuitive mind, it will be found that a great harmony has begun to lay its own foundations. This harmony will be other than that created by the intellectual mind and indeed may not be easily perceptible or, if it is felt, yet not intelligible to the logical man, because not arrived at or analysable by his mental process. It will be a harmony of the spontaneous expression of the spirit.

As soon as we arise above mind to the supermind, this initial harmony will be replaced by a greater and a more integral unity. The thoughts of the supramental reason meet together and understand each other and fall into a natural arrangement even when they have started from quite opposite quarters. The movements of will that are in conflict in the mind, come in the supermind to their right place and relation to each other. The supramental feelings also discover their own affinities and fall into a natural agreement and harmony. At a higher stage this harmony intensifies towards unity. The knowledge, will, feeling and all else become a single movement. This unity reaches its greatest completeness in the highest supermind. The harmony, the unity are inevitable because the base in the supermind is knowledge and characteristically self-knowledge, the knowledge of the self in all its aspects. The supramental will is the dynamic expression of this self-knowledge, the supramental feeling the expression of the luminous joy of the self and all else in supermind a part of this one movement. At its highest range it becomes something greater than what we call knowledge; there it is the essential and integral self-awareness of the Divine in us, his being, consciousness, Tapas, Ananda, and all is the harmonious, unified, luminous movement of that one existence.

This supramental knowledge is not primarily or essentially a thought knowledge. The intellect does not consider that it knows a thing until it has reduced its awareness of it to the terms of thought, not, that is to say, until it has put it into a system of representative mental concepts, and this kind of knowledge gets its most decisive completeness when it can be put into clear, precise and defining speech. It is true that the mind gets its knowledge primarily by various kinds of impression beginning from the vital and the sense impressions and rising to the intuitive, but these are taken by the developed intelligence only as data and seem to it uncertain and vague in themselves until they have been forced to yield up all their content to the thought and have taken their place in some intellectual relation or in an ordered thought sequence. It is true again that there is a thought and a speech which are rather suggestive than definitive and have in their own way a greater potency and richness of content, and this kind already verges on the intuitive: but still there is a demand in the intellect to bring out in clear sequence and relation the exact intellectual content of these suggestions and until that is done it does not feel satisfied that its knowledge is complete. The thought labouring in the logical intellect is that which normally seems best to organise the mental action and gives to the mind a sense of sure definiteness, security and completeness in its knowledge and its use of knowledge. Nothing of this is at all true of the supramental knowledge.

The supermind knows most completely and securely not by thought but by identity, by a pure awareness of the self-truth of things in the self and by the self, *ātmani ātmānam ātmanā*. I get the supramental knowledge best by becoming one with the truth, one with the object of knowledge; the supramental satisfaction and integral light is most there when there is no further division between the knower, knowledge and the known, *jñātā, jñānam, jñeyam*. I see the thing known not as an object outside myself, but as myself or a part of my universal self contained in my most direct consciousness. This leads to the highest and completest knowledge; thought and speech being representations and not this direct possession in the consciousness are to the supermind a lesser form and, if not filled with the spiritual awareness, thought becomes in fact a diminution of knowledge. For it would be, supposing it to be a supramental thought, only a partial manifestation of a greater knowledge existing in the self but not at the time present to the immediately active consciousness. In the highest ranges of the infinite there need be no thought at all because all would be experienced spiritually, in continuity, in eternal possession and with an absolute directness and completeness. Thought is only one means of partially manifesting and presenting what is hidden in this greater self-existent knowledge. This supreme kind of knowing will not indeed be possible to us in its full extent and degree until we can rise through many grades of the supermind to that infinite. But still as the supramental power emerges and enlarges its action, something of this highest way of knowledge appears and grows and even the members of the mental being, as they are intuitivised and supramentalised, develop more and more a corresponding action upon their own level. There is an increasing power of a luminous vital, psychic, emotional, dynamic and other identification with all the things and beings that are the objects of our consciousness and these transcendings of the separative consciousness bring with them many forms and means of a direct knowledge.

The supramental knowledge or experience by identity carries in it as a result or as a secondary part of itself a supramental vision that needs the support of no image, can concretise what is to the mind abstract and has the character of sight though its object may be the invisible truth of that which has form or the truth of the formless. This vision can come before there is any identity, as a sort of previous emanation of light from it, or may act detached from it as a separate power. The truth or the thing known is then not altogether or not yet one with myself, but an object of my knowledge: but still it is an object subjectively seen in the self or at least, even if it is still farther separated and objectivised to the knower, by the self, not through any intermediate process, but by a direct inner seizing or a penetrating and enveloping luminous contact of the spiritual consciousness with its object. It is this luminous seizing and contact that is the spiritual vision, *dṛṣṭi*,—"*paśyati*", says the Upanishad continually of the spiritual knowledge, "he sees"; and of the Self conceiving the idea of creation, where we should expect "he thought", it says instead "he saw". It is to the spirit what the eyes are to the physical mind and one has the sense of having passed through a subtly analogous process. As the physical sight can present to us the actual body of things of which the thought had only possessed an indication or mental description and they become to us at once real and evident, *pratyakṣa*, so the spiritual sight surpasses the indications or representations of thought and can make the self and truth of all things present to us and directly evident, *pratyakṣa*.

The sense can only give us the superficial image of things and it needs the aid of thought to fill and inform the image; but the spiritual sight is capable of presenting to us the thing in itself and all truth about it. The seer does not need the aid of thought in its process as a means of knowledge, but only as a means of representation and expression,— thought is to him a lesser power and used for a secondary purpose. If a further extension of knowledge is required, he can come at it by new seeing without the slower thought processes that are the staff of support of the mental search and its feeling out for truth,—even as we scrutinise with the eye to find what escaped our first observation. This experience and knowledge by spiritual vision is the second in directness and greatness of the supramental powers. It is something much more near, profound and comprehensive than mental vision, because it derives direct from the knowledge by identity, and it has this virtue that we can proceed at once from the vision to the identity, as from the identity to the vision. Thus when the spiritual vision has seen God, Self or Brahman, the soul can next enter into and become one with the Self, God or Brahman.

This can only be done integrally on or above the supramental level, but at the same time the spiritual vision can take on mental forms of itself that can help towards this identification each in its own way. A mental intuitive vision or a spiritualised mental sight, a psychic vision, an emotional vision of the heart, a vision in the sense mind are parts of the Yogic experience. If these seeings are purely mental, then they may but need not be true, for the mind is capable of both truth and error, both of a true and of a false representation. But as the mind becomes intuitivised and supramentalised, these powers are purified and corrected by the more luminous action of the supermind and become themselves forms of a supramental and a true seeing. The supramental vision, it may be noted, brings with it a supplementary and completing experience that might be called a spiritual hearing and touch of the truth,—of its essence and through that of its significance,—that is to say, there is a seizing of its movement, vibration, rhythm and a seizing of its close presence and contact and substance. All these powers prepare us to become one with that which has thus grown near to us through knowledge.

The supramental thought is a form of the knowledge by identity and a development, in the idea, of the truth presented to the supramental vision. The identity and the vision give the truth in its essence, its body and its parts in a single view: the thought translates this direct consciousness and immediate power of the truth into idea-knowledge and will. It adds or need add otherwise nothing new, but reproduces, articulates, moves round the body of the knowledge. Where, however, the identity and the vision are still incomplete, the supramental thought has a larger office and reveals, interprets or recalls as it were to the soul's memory what they are not yet ready to give. And where these greater states and powers are still veiled, the thought comes in front and prepares and to a certain extent effects a partial rending or helps actively in the removal of the veil. Therefore in the development out of the mental ignorance into the supramental knowledge this illumined thought comes to us often though not always first, to open the way to the vision or else to give first supports to the growing consciousness of identity and its greater knowledge. This thought is also an effective means of communication and expression and helps to an impression or fixation of the truth whether on one's own lower mind and being or on that of others. The supramental thought differs from the intellectual not only because it is the direct truth idea and not a representation of truth to the ignorance,—it is the truth consciousness of the spirit always presenting to itself its own right forms, the *satyam* and *ṛtam* of the Veda,—but because of its strong reality, body of light and substance.

The intellectual thought refines and sublimates to a rarefied abstractness; the supramental thought as it rises in its height increases to a greater spiritual concreteness. The thought of the intellect presents itself to us as an abstraction from something seized by the mind sense and is as if supported in a void and subtle air of mind by an intangible force of the intelligence. It has to resort to a use of the mind's power of image if it wishes to make itself more concretely felt and seen by the soul sense and soul vision. The supramental thought on the contrary presents always the idea as a luminous substance of being, luminous stuff of consciousness taking significative thought form and it therefore creates no such sense of a gulf between the idea and the real as we are liable to feel in the mind, but is itself a reality, it is real-idea and the body of a reality. It has as a result, associated with it when it acts according to its own nature, a phenomenon of spiritual light other than the intellectual clarity, a great realising force and a luminous ecstasy. It is an intensely sensible vibration of being, consciousness and Ananda.

The supramental thought, as has already been indicated, has three elevations of its intensity, one of direct thought vision, another of interpretative vision pointing to and preparing the greater revelatory idea-sight, a third of representative vision recalling as it were to the spirit's knowledge the truth that is called out more directly by the higher powers. In the mind these things take the form of the three ordinary powers of the intuitive mentality,—the suggestive and discriminating intuition, the inspiration and the thought that is of the nature of revelation. Above they correspond to three elevations of the supramental being and consciousness and, as we ascend, the lower first calls down into itself and is then taken up into the higher, so that on each level all the three elevations are reproduced, but always there predominates in the thought essence the character that belongs to that level's proper form of consciousness and spiritual substance. It is necessary to bear this in mind; for otherwise the mentality, looking up to the ranges of the supermind as they reveal themselves, may think it has got the vision of the highest heights when it is only the highest range of the lower ascent that is being presented to its experience. At each height, *sānoḥ sānum āruhat*, the powers of the supermind increase in intensity, range and completeness.

There is also a speech, a supramental word, in which the higher knowledge, vision or thought can clothe itself within us for expression. At first this may come down as a word, a message or an inspiration that descends to us from above or it may even seem a voice of the Self or of the Ishwara, *vāṇī, ādeśa*. Afterwards it loses that separate character and becomes the normal form of the thought when it expresses itself in the form of an inward speech. The thought may express itself without the aid of any suggestive or developing word and only—but still quite completely, explicitly and with its full contents—in a luminous substance of supramental perception. It may aid itself when it is not so explicit by a suggestive inward speech that attends it to bring out its whole significance. Or the thought may come not as silent perception but as speech self-born out of the truth and complete in its own right and carrying in itself its own vision and knowledge. Then it is the word revelatory, inspired or intuitive or of a yet greater kind capable of bearing the infinite intention or suggestion of the higher supermind and spirit. It may frame itself in the language now employed to express the ideas and perceptions and impulses of the intellect and the sense mind, but it uses it in a different way and with an intense bringing out of the intuitive or revelatory significances of which speech is capable. The supramental word manifests inwardly with a light, a power, a rhythm of thought and a rhythm of inner sound that make it the natural and living body of the supramental thought and vision and it pours into the language, even though the same as that of mental speech, another than the limited intellectual, emotional or sensational significance. It is formed and heard in the intuitive mind or supermind and need not at first except in certain highly gifted souls come out easily into speech and writing, but that too can be freely done when the physical consciousness and its organs have been made ready, and this is a part of the needed fullness and power of the integral perfection.

The range of knowledge covered by the supramental thought, experience and vision will be commensurate with all that is open to the human consciousness, not only on the earthly but on all planes. It will however act increasingly in an inverse sense to that of the mental thinking and experience. The centre of mental thinking is the ego, the person of the individual thinker. The supramental man on the contrary will think more with the universal mind or even may rise above it, and his individuality will rather be a vessel of radiation and communication to which the universal thought and knowledge of the Spirit will converge than a centre. The mental man thinks and acts in a radius determined by the smallness or largeness of his mentality and of its experience. The range of the supramental man will be all the earth and all that lies behind it on other planes of existence. And finally the mental man thinks and sees on the level of the present life, though it may be with an upward aspiration, and his view is obstructed on every side. His main basis of knowledge and action is the present with a glimpse into the past and ill-grasped influence from its pressure and a blind look towards the future. He bases himself on the actualities of the earthly existence, first on the facts of the outward world,—to which he is ordinarily in the habit of relating nine tenths if not the whole of his inner thinking and experience,—then on the changing actualities of the more superficial part of his inner being. As he increases in mind, he goes more freely beyond these to potentialities which arise out of them and pass beyond them; his mind deals with a larger field of possibilities: but these for the most part get to him a full reality only in proportion as they are related to the actual and can be made actual here, now or hereafter. The essence of things he tends to see, if at all, only as a result of his actualities, in a relation to and dependence on them, and therefore he sees them constantly in a false light or in a limited measure. In all these respects the supramental man must proceed from the opposite principle of truth vision.

The supramental being sees things from above in large spaces and at the highest from the spaces of the infinite. His view is not limited to the standpoint of the present but can see in the continuities of time or from above time in the indivisibilities of the Spirit. He sees truth in its proper order first in the essence, secondly in the potentialities that derive from it and only last in the actualities. The essential truths are to his sight self-existent, self-seen, not dependent for their proof on this or that actuality; the potential truths are truths of the power of being in itself and in things, truths of the infinity of force and real apart from their past or present realisation in this or that actuality or the habitual surface forms that we take for the whole of Nature; the actualities are only a selection from the potential truths he sees, dependent on them, limited and mutable. The tyranny of the present, of the actual, of the immediate range of facts, of the immediate urge and demand of action has no power over his thought and his will and he is therefore able to have a larger will-power founded on a larger knowledge. He sees things not as one on the levels surrounded by the jungle of present facts and phenomena but from above, not from outside and judged by their surfaces, but from within and viewed from the truth of their centre; therefore he is nearer the divine omniscience. He wills and acts from a dominating height and with a longer movement in time and a larger range of potencies, therefore he is nearer to the divine omnipotence. His being is not shut into the succession of the moments, but has the full power of the past and ranges seeingly through the future: not shut in the limiting ego and personal mind, but lives in the freedom of the universal, in God and in all beings and all things; not in the dull density of the physical mind, but in the light of the self and the infinity of the spirit. He sees soul and mind only as a power and a movement and matter only as a resultant form of the spirit. All his thought will be of a kind that proceeds from knowledge. He perceives and enacts the things of the phenomenal life in the light of the reality of the spiritual being and the power of the dynamic spiritual essence.

At first, at the beginning of the conversion into this greater status, the thought will continue to move for a shorter or a longer time to a greater or a less extent on the lines of the mind but with a greater light and increasing flights and spaces and movements of freedom and transcendence. Afterwards the freedom and transcendence will begin to predominate; the inversion of the thought view and the conversion of the thought method will take place in different movements of the thought mind one after the other, subject to whatever difficulties and relapses, until it has gained on the whole and effected a complete transformation. Ordinarily the supramental knowledge will be organised first and with the most ease in the processes of pure thought and knowledge, *jñāna*, because here the human mind has already the upward tendency and is the most free. Next and with less ease it will be organised in the processes of applied thought and knowledge because there the mind of man is at once most active and most bound and wedded to its inferior methods. The last and most difficult conquest, because this is now to his mind a field of conjecture or a blank, will be the knowledge of the three times, *trikāladṛṣṭi*. In all these there will be the same character of a spirit seeing and willing directly above and around and not only in the body it possesses and there will be the same action of the supramental knowledge by identity, the supramental vision, the supramental thought and supramental word, separately or in a united movement.

This then will be the general character of the supramental thought and knowledge and these its main powers and action. It remains to consider its particular instrumentation, the change that the supermind will make in the different elements of the present human mentality and the special activities that give to the thought its constituents, motives and data.

# THE SUPRAMENTAL INSTRUMENTS — THOUGHT-PROCESS

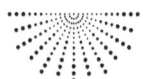

THE SUPERMIND, the divine gnosis, is not something entirely alien to our present consciousness: it is a superior instrumentation of the spirit and all the operations of our normal consciousness are limited and inferior derivations from the supramental, because these are tentatives and constructions, that the true and perfect, the spontaneous and harmonious nature and action of the spirit. Accordingly when we rise from mind to supermind, the new power of consciousness does not reject, but uplifts, enlarges and transfigures the operations of our soul and mind and life. It exalts and gives to them an ever greater reality of their power and performance. It does not limit itself either to the transformation of the superficial powers and action of the mind and psychic parts and the life, but it manifests and transforms also those rarer powers and that larger force and knowledge proper to our subliminal self that appear now to us as things occult, curiously psychic, abnormal. These things become in the supramental nature not at all abnormal but perfectly natural and normal, not separately psychic but spiritual, not occult and strange, but a direct, simple, inherent and spontaneous action. The spirit is not limited like the waking material consciousness, and the supermind when it takes possession of the waking consciousness, dematerialises it, delivers it from its limits, converts the material and the psychic into the nature of the spiritual being.

The mental activity that can be most readily organised is, as has been already indicated, that of pure ideative knowledge. This is transformed on the higher level to the true *jñāna*, supramental thought, supramental vision, the supramental knowledge by identity. The essential action of this supramental knowledge has been described in the preceding chapter. It is necessary however to see also how this knowledge works in outward application and how it deals with the data of existence. It differs from the action of the mind first in this respect that it works naturally with those operations that are to the mind the highest and the most difficult, acting in them or on them from above downward and not with the hampered straining upward of the mind or with its restriction to its own and the inferior levels. The higher operations are not dependent on the lower assistance, but rather the lower operations depend on the higher not only for their guidance but for their existence. The lower mental operations are therefore not only changed in character by the transformation, but are made entirely subordinate. And the higher mental operations too change their character, because, supramentalised, they begin to derive their light directly from the highest, the self-knowledge or infinite knowledge.

The normal thought-action of the mind may for this purpose be viewed as constituted of a triple motion. First and lowest and most necessary to the mental being in the body is the habitual thought mind that founds its ideas upon the data given by the senses and by the surface experiences of the nervous and emotional being and on the customary notions formed by the education and the outward life and environment. This habitual mind has two movements, one a kind of constant undercurrent of mechanically recurrent thought always repeating itself in the same round of physical, vital, emotional, practical and summarily intellectual notion and experience, the other more actively working upon all new experience that the mind is obliged to admit and reducing it to formulas of habitual thinking. The mentality of the average man is limited by this habitual mind and moves very imperfectly outside its circle.

A second grade of the thinking activity is the pragmatic idea mind that lifts itself above life and acts creatively as a mediator between the idea and the life-power, between truth of life and truth of the idea not yet manifested in life. It draws material from life and builds out of it and upon it creative ideas that become dynamic for farther life development: on the other side it receives new thought and mental experience from the mental plane or more fundamentally from the idea power of the Infinite and immediately turns it into mental idea force and a power for actual being and living. The whole turn of this pragmatic idea mind is towards action and experience, inward as well as outward, the inward casting itself outward for the sake of a completer satisfaction of reality, the outward taken into the inward and returning upon it assimilated and changed for fresh formations. The thought is only or mainly interesting to the soul on this mental level as a means for a large range of action and experience.

A third gradation of thinking opens in us the pure ideative mind which lives disinterestedly in truth of the idea apart from any necessary dependence on its value for action and experience. It views the data of the senses and the superficial inner experience, but only to find the idea, the truth to which they bear witness and to reduce them into terms of knowledge. It observes the creative action of mind in life in the same way and for the same purpose. Its preoccupation is with knowledge, its whole object is to have the delight of ideation, the search for truth, the effort to know itself and the world and all that may lie behind its own action and the world action. This ideative mind is the highest reach of the intellect acting for itself, characteristically, in its own power and for its own purpose.

It is difficult for the human mind to combine rightly and harmonise these three movements of the intelligence. The ordinary man lives mainly in the habitual, has a comparatively feeble action of the creative and pragmatic and experiences a great difficulty in using at all or entering into the movement of the pure ideative mentality. The creative pragmatic mind is commonly too much occupied with its own motion to move freely and disinterestedly in the atmosphere of pure ideative order and on the other hand has often an insufficient grasp on the actualities imposed by the habitual mentality and the obstacles it imposes as also on other movements of pragmatic thought and action than that which it is itself interested in building. The pure ideative mentality tends to construct abstract and arbitrary systems of truth, intellectual sections and ideative edifices, and either misses the pragmatic movement necessary to life and lives only or mainly in ideas, or cannot act with sufficient power and directness in the life field and is in danger of being divorced from or weak in the world of the practical and habitual mentality. An accommodation of some kind is made, but the tyranny of the predominant tendency interferes with the wholeness and unity of the thinking being.

Mind fails to be assured master even of its own totality, because the secret of that totality lies beyond it in the free unity of the self, free and therefore capable of an infinite multiplicity and diversity, and in the supramental power that can alone bring out in a natural perfection the organic multiple movement of the self's unity.

The supermind in its completeness reverses the whole order of the mind's thinking. It lives not in the phenomenal, but in the essential, in the self, and sees all as being of the self and its power and form and movement, and all the thought and the process of the thought in the supermind must also be of that character. All its fundamental ideation is a rendering of the spiritual knowledge that acts by identity with all being and of the supramental vision. It moves therefore primarily among the eternal, the essential and the universal truths of self and being and consciousness and infinite power and delight of being (not excluding all that seems to our present consciousness non-being), and all its particular thinking originates from and depends upon the power of these eternal verities; but in the second place it is at home too with infinite aspects and applications, sequences and harmonies of the truths of being of the Eternal. It lives therefore at its heights in all that which the action of the pure ideative mind is an effort to reach and discover, and even on its lower ranges these things are to its luminous receptivity present, near or easily grasped and available.

But while the highest truths or the pure ideas are to the ideative mind abstractions, because mind lives partly in the phenomenal and partly in intellectual constructions and has to use the method of abstraction to arrive at the higher realities, the supermind lives in the spirit and therefore in the very substance of what these ideas and truths represent or rather fundamentally are and truly realises them, not only thinks but in the act of thinking feels and identifies itself with their substance, and to it they are among the most substantial things that can be. Truths of consciousness and of essential being are to the supermind the very stuff of reality, more intimately and, as one might almost say, densely real than outward movement and form of being, although these too are to it movement and form of the reality and not, as they are to a certain action of the spiritualised mind, an illusion. The idea too is to it real-idea, stuff of the reality of conscious being, full of power for the substantial rendering of the truth and therefore for creation.

And again, while the pure ideative mind tends to build up arbitrary systems which are mental and partial constructions of the truth, the supermind is not bound by any representation or system, though it is perfectly able to represent and to arrange and construct in the living substance of the truth for the pragmatic purposes of the Infinite. The mind when it gets free from its exclusivenesses, systematising, attachment to its own constructions, is at a loss in the infiniteness of the infinite, feels it as a chaos, even if a luminous chaos, is unable any longer to formulate and therefore to think and act decisively because all, even the most diverse or contradictory things, point at some truth in this infinity and yet nothing it can think is entirely true and all its formulations break down under the test of new suggestions from the infinite. It begins to look on the world as a phantasmagory and thought as a chaos of scintillations out of the luminous indefinite. The mind assailed by the vastness and freedom of the supramental loses itself and finds no firm footing in the vastness. The supermind on the contrary can in its freedom construct harmonies of its thought and expression of being on the firm ground of reality while still holding its infinite liberty and rejoicing in its self of infinite vastness. All that it thinks, as all that it is and does and lives, belongs to the truth, the right, the vast, *satyam, ṛtam, bṛhat*.

The result of this wholeness is that there is no division or incompatibility between the free essential ideation of the supermind corresponding to the mind's pure ideation, free, disinterested, illimitable, and its creative, pragmatic ideation purposeful and determinative. The infinity of being results naturally in a freedom of the harmonies of becoming. The supermind perceives always action as a manifestation and expression of the Self and creation as a revelation of the Infinite. All its creative and pragmatic thought is an instrument of the self's becoming, a power of illumination for that purpose, an intermediary between the eternal identity and infinite novelty and variety of illimitable Being and its self-expression in the worlds and life. It is this that the supermind constantly sees and embodies and while its ideative vision and thought interpret to it the illimitable unity and variety of the Infinite, which it is by a perpetual identity and in which it lives in all its power of being and becoming, there is constantly too a special creative thought, associated with an action of the infinite will, Tapas, power of being, which determines what it shall present, manifest or create out of the infinite in the course of Time, what it shall make—here and now or in any range of Time or world—of the perpetual becoming of the self in the universe.

The supermind is not limited by this pragmatic movement and does not take the partial motion or the entire stream of what it so becomes and creates in its thought and life for the whole truth of its self or of the Infinite. It does not live only in what it is and thinks and does selectively in the present or on one plane only of being; it does not feed its existence only on the present or the continual succession of moments to whose beats we give that name. It does not see itself only as a movement of Time or of the consciousness in time or as a creature of the perpetual becoming. It is aware of a timeless being beyond manifestation and of which all is a manifestation, it is aware of what is eternal even in Time, it is aware of many planes of existence; it is aware of past truth of manifestation and of much truth of being yet to be manifested in the future, but already existing in the self-view of the Eternal. It does not mistake the pragmatic reality which is the truth of action and mutation for the sole truth, but sees it as a constant realisation of that which is eternally real. It knows that creation whether on the plane of matter or of life or of mind or of supermind is and can be only a self-determined presentation of eternal truth, a revelation of the Eternal, and it is intimately aware of the pre-existence of the truth of all things in the Eternal. This seeing conditions all its pragmatic thought and its resultant action. The maker in it is a selective power of the seer and thinker, the self-builder a power of the self-seer, the self-expressing soul a power of the infinite spirit. It creates freely, and all the more surely and decisively for that freedom, out of the infinite self and spirit.

It is therefore not prisoned in its special becoming or shut up in its round or its course of action. It is open, in a way and a degree to which the mind cannot attain, to the truth of other harmonies of creative becoming even while in its own it puts forth a decisive will and thought and action. When it is engaged in action that is of the nature of a struggle, the replacing of past or other thought and form and becoming by that which it is appointed to manifest, it knows the truth of what it displaces and fulfils even in displacing as well as the truth of what it substitutes. It is not bound by its manifesting, selecting, pragmatic conscious action, but it has at the same time all the joy of a specially creative thought and selective precision of action, the Ananda of the truth of the forms and movements equally of its own and of others' becoming. All its thought and will of life and action and creation, rich, manifold, focussing the truth of many planes, is liberated and illumined with the illimitable truth of the Eternal.

This creative or pragmatic movement of the supramental thought and consciousness brings with it an action which corresponds to that of the habitual or mechanical mentality but is yet of a very different character. The thing that is created is the self-determination of a harmony and all harmony proceeds upon seen or given lines and carries with it a constant pulsation and rhythmic recurrence. The supramental thought, organising the harmony of manifested existence of the supramental being, founds it on eternal principles, casts it upon the right lines of the truth that is to be manifested, keeps sounding as characteristic notes the recurrence of the constant elements in the experience and the action which are necessary to constitute the harmony. There is an order of the thought, a cycle of the will, a stability in the motion. At the same time its freedom prevents it from being shut up by the recurrence into a groove of habitual action turning always mechanically round a limited stock of thinking. It does not like the habitual mind refer and assimilate all new thought and experience to a fixed customary mould of thinking, taking that for its basis. Its basis, that to which all is referred, is above, *upari budhne*, in the largeness of the self, in the supreme foundation of the supramental truth, *budhne ṛtasya*. Its order of thought, its cycle of will, its stable movement of action does not crystallise into a mechanism or convention, but is always alive with the spirit, does not live by exclusiveness or hostility to other coexistent or possible order and cycle, but absorbs sustenance from all that it contacts and assimilates it to its own principle. The spiritual assimilation is practicable because all is referred to the largeness of the self and its free vision above. The order of the supramental thought and will is constantly receiving new light and power from above and has no difficulty in accepting it into its movement; it is, as is proper to an order of the Infinite, even in its stability of motion indescribably supple and plastic, capable of perceiving and rendering the relation of all things to each other in the One, capable of expressing always more and more of the Infinite, at its fullest of expressing in its own way all that is actually expressible of the Infinite.

Thus there is no discord, disparity or difficulty of adjustment in the complex motion of the supramental *jñ ā na*, but a simplicity in the complexity, an assured ease in a many-sided abundance that comes from the spontaneous sureness and totality of the self-knowledge of the spirit. Obstacle, inner struggle, disparity, difficulty, discord of parts and movements continues in the transformation of mind to supermind only so long as the action, influence or pressure of the mind insisting on its own methods of construction continues or its process of building knowledge or thought and will of action on the foundation of a primal ignorance resists the opposite process of supermind organising all as a luminous manifestation out of the self and its inherent and eternal self-knowledge. It is thus that the supermind acting as a representative, interpretative, revealingly imperative power of the spirit's knowledge by identity, turning the light of the infinite consciousness freely and illimitably into substance and form of real-idea, creating out of power of conscious being and power of real-idea, stabilising a movement which obeys its own law but is still a supple and plastic movement of the infinite, uses its thought and knowledge and a will identical in substance and light with the knowledge to organise in each supramental being his own right manifestation of the one self and spirit.

The action of the supramental *jñāna* so constituted evidently surpasses the action of the mental reason and we have to see what replaces the reason in the supramental transformation. The thinking mind of man finds its most clear and characteristic satisfaction and its most precise and effective principle of organisation in the reasoning and logical intelligence. It is true that man is not and cannot be wholly governed either in his thought or his action by the reason alone. His mentality is inextricably subjected to a joint, mixed and intricate action of the reasoning intelligence with two other powers, an intuition, actually only half luminous in the human mentality, operating behind the more visible action of the reason or veiled and altered in the action of the normal intelligence, and the life-mind of sensation, instinct, impulse, which is in its own nature a sort of obscure involved intuition and which supplies the intelligence from below with its first materials and data. And each of these other powers is in its own kind an intimate action of the spirit operating in mind and life and has a more direct and spontaneous character and immediate power for perception and action than the reasoning intelligence. But yet neither of these powers is capable of organising for man his mental existence.

His life-mind—its instincts, its impulses,—is not and cannot be self-sufficient and predominant as it is in the lower creation. It has been seized upon by the intelligence and profoundly altered by it even where the development of the intelligence is imperfect and itself most insistent in its prominence. It has lost most of its intuitive character, is indeed now infinitely richer as a supplier of materials and data, but no longer quite itself or at ease in its action because half rationalised, dependent at least on some infused element however vague of reasoning or intelligent activity and incapable of acting to good purpose without the aid of the intelligence. Its roots and place of perfection are in the subconscient from which it emerges and man's business is to increase in the sense of a more and more conscient knowledge and action. Man reverting to a governance of his being by the life mind would become either irrational and erratic or dull and imbecile and would lose the essential character of manhood.

The intuition on the other hand has its roots and its place of perfection in the supramental which is now to us the superconscient, and in mind it has no pure and no organised action, but is immediately mixed with the action of the reasoning intelligence, is not quite itself, but limited, fragmentary, diluted and impure, and depends for the ordered use and organisation of its suggestions on the aid of the logical reason. The human mind is never quite sure of its intuitions until they have been viewed and confirmed by the judgment of the rational intelligence: it is there that it feels most well founded and secure. Man surmounting reason to organise his thought and life by the intuitive mind would be already surpassing his characteristic humanity and on the way to the development of supermanhood. This can only be done above: for to attempt it below is only to achieve another kind of imperfection: there the mental reason is a necessary factor.

The reasoning intelligence is an intermediate agent between the life mind and the yet undeveloped supramental intuition. Its business is that of an intermediary, on the one side to enlighten the life mind, to make it conscient and govern and regulate as much as may be its action until Nature is ready to evolve the supramental energy which will take hold of life and illumine and perfect all its movements by converting its obscurely intuitive motions of desire, emotion, sensation and action into a spiritually and luminously spontaneous life manifestation of the self and spirit. On the other higher side its mission is to take the rays of light which come from above and translate them into terms of intelligent mentality and to accept, examine, develop, intellectually utilise the intuitions that escape the barrier and descend into mind from the superconscience. It does this until man, becoming more and more intelligently conscient of himself and his environment and his being, becomes also aware that he cannot really know these things by his reason, but can only make a mental representation of them to his intelligence.

The reason, however, tends in the intellectual man to ignore the limitations of its power and function and attempts to be not an instrument and agent but a substitute for the self and spirit. Made confident by success and predominance, by the comparative greatness of its own light, it regards itself as a thing primary and absolute, assures itself of its own entire truth and sufficiency and endeavours to become the absolute ruler of mind and life. This it cannot do successfully, because it depends on the lower life intuition and on the covert supermind and its intuitive messages for its own real substance and existence. It can only appear to itself to succeed because it reduces all its experience to rational formulas and blinds itself to half the real nature of the thought and action that is behind it and to the infinite deal that breaks out of its formulas. The excess of the reason only makes life artificial and rationally mechanical, deprives it of its spontaneity and vitality and prevents the freedom and expansion of the spirit. The limited and limiting mental reason must make itself plastic and flexible, open itself to its source, receive the light from above, exceed itself and pass by an euthanasia of transformation into the body of the supramental reason. Meanwhile it is given power and leading for an organisation of thought and action on the characteristically human scale intermediate between the subconscient power of the spirit organising the life of the animal and the superconscient power of the spirit which becoming conscient can organise the existence and life of a spiritual supermanhood.

The characteristic power of the reason in its fullness is a logical movement assuring itself first of all available materials and data by observation and arrangement, then acting upon them for a resultant knowledge gained, assured and enlarged by a first use of the reflective powers, and lastly assuring itself of the correctness of its results by a more careful and formal action, more vigilant, deliberate, severely logical which tests, rejects or confirms them according to certain secure standards and processes developed by reflection and experience. The first business of the logical reason is therefore a right, careful and complete observation of its available material and data. The first and easiest field of data open to our knowledge is the world of Nature, of the physical objects made external to it by the separative action of mind, things not ourself and therefore only indirectly knowable by an interpreting of our sense perceptions, by observation, accumulated experience, inference and reflective thinking. Another field is our own internal being and its movements which one knows naturally by an internally acting mental sense by intuitive perception and constant experience and by reflective thought on the evidences of our nature. The reason with regard even to these inner movements acts best and knows them most correctly by detaching itself and regarding them quite impersonally and objectively, a movement which in the Yoga of knowledge ends in viewing our own active being too as not self, a mechanism of Nature like the rest of the world-existence. The knowledge of other thinking and conscious beings stands between these two fields, but is gained, too, indirectly by observation, by experience, by various means of communication and, acting on these, by reflection and inference largely founded on analogy from our knowledge of our own nature. Another field of data which the reason has to observe is its own action and the action of the whole human intelligence, for without that study it cannot be assured of the correctness of its knowledge or of right method and process. Finally, there are other fields of knowledge for which the data are not so easily available and which need the development of abnormal faculties,—the discovery of things and ranges of existence behind the appearances of the physical world and the discovery of the secret self or principle of being of man and of Nature. The first the logical reason can attempt to deal with, accepting subject to its scrutiny whatever data become available, in the same way as it deals with the physical world, but ordinarily it is little disposed to deal with them, finding it more easy to question and deny, and its action here is seldom assured or effective. The second it usually attempts to discover by a constructive metaphysical logic founded on its analytic and synthetic observation of the phenomena of life, mind and matter.

The operation of the logical reason is the same in all these fields of its data. At first the intelligence amasses a store of observations, associations, percepts, recepts, concepts, makes a more or less obvious arrangement and classification of relations and of things according to their likenesses and differences, and works upon them by an accumulating store and a constant addition of ideas, memories, imaginations, judgments; these make up primarily the nature of activity of our knowledge. There is a kind of natural enlargement of this intelligent activity of the mind progressing by its own momentum, an evolution aided more and more by a deliberate culture, the increase of faculties gained by the culture becoming in its turn a part of the nature as they settle into a more spontaneous action,—the result a progression not of the character and essential power of the intelligence, but of its degree of power, flexibility, variety of capacity, fineness. There is a correction of errors, an accumulating of assured ideas and judgments, a reception or formation of fresh knowledge. At the same time a necessity arises for a more precise and assured action of the intelligence which will get rid of the superficiality of this ordinary method of the intelligence, test every step, scrutinise severely every conclusion and reduce the mind's action to a well-founded system and order.

This movement develops the complete logical mind and raises to its acme the acuteness and power of the intelligence. The rougher and more superficial observation is replaced or supplemented by a scrutinising analysis of all the process, properties, constituents, energies making up or related to the object and a synthetic construction of it as a whole which is added to or in great part substituted for the mind's natural conception of it. The object is more precisely distinguished from all others and at the same time there is a completer discovery of its relations with others. There is a fixing of sameness or likeness and kinship and also of divergences and differences resulting on one side in the perception of the fundamental unity of being and Nature and the similarity and continuity of their processes, on the other in a clear precision and classification of different energies and kinds of beings and objects. The amassing and ordering of the materials and data of knowledge are carried to perfection as far as is possible to the logical intelligence.

Memory is the indispensable aid of the mind to preserve its past observations, the memory of the individual but also of the race, whether in the artificial form of accumulated records or the general race memory preserving its gains with a sort of constant repetition and renewal and, an element not sufficiently appreciated, a latent memory that can under the pressure of various kinds of stimulation repeat under new conditions past movements of knowledge for judgment by the increased information and intelligence. The developed logical mind puts into order the action and resources of the human memory and trains it to make the utmost use of its materials. The human judgment naturally works on these materials in two ways, by a more or less rapid and summary combination of observation, inference, creative or critical conclusion, insight, immediate idea—this is largely an attempt of the mind to work in a spontaneous manner with the directness that can only be securely achieved by the higher faculty of the intuition, for in the mind it produces much false confidence and unreliable certitude,—and a slower but in the end intellectually surer seeking, considering and testing judgment that develops into the careful logical action.

The memory and judgment are both aided by the imagination which, as a function of knowledge, suggests possibilities not actually presented or justified by the other powers and opens the doors to fresh vistas. The developed logical intelligence uses the imagination for suggesting new discovery and hypothesis, but is careful to test its suggestions fully by observation and a sceptical or scrupulous judgment. It insists too on testing, as far as may be, all the action of the judgment itself, rejects hasty inference in favour of an ordered system of deduction and induction and makes sure of all its steps and of the justice, continuity, compatibility, cohesion of its conclusions. A too formalised logical mind discourages, but a free use of the whole action of the logical intelligence may rather heighten a certain action of immediate insight, the mind's nearest approach to the higher intuition, but it does not place on it an unqualified reliance. The endeavour of the logical reason is always by a detached, disinterested and carefully founded method to get rid of error, of prejudgment, of the mind's false confidence and arrive at reliable certitudes.

And if this elaborated method of the mind were really sufficient for truth, there would be no need of any higher step in the evolution of knowledge. In fact, it increases the mind's hold on itself and on the world around it and serves great and undeniable utilities: but it can never be sure whether its data supply it with the frame of a real knowledge or only a frame useful and necessary for the human mind and will in its own present form of action. It is more and more perceived that the knowledge of phenomena increases, but the knowledge of reality escapes this laborious process. A time must come, is already coming when the mind perceives the necessity of calling to its aid and developing fully the intuition and all the great range of powers that lie concealed behind our vague use of the word and uncertain perception of its significance. In the end it must discover that these powers cannot only aid and complete but even replace its own proper action. That will be the beginning of the discovery of the supramental energy of the spirit.

The supermind, as we have seen, lifts up the action of the mental consciousness towards and into the intuition, creates an intermediate intuitive mentality insufficient in itself but greater in power than the logical intelligence, and then lifts up and transforms that too into the true supramental action. The first well-organised action of the supermind in the ascending order is the supramental reason, not a higher logical intellect, but a directly luminous organisation of intimately subjective and intimately objective knowledge, the higher *buddhi*, the logical or rather the logos Vijnana. The supramental reason does all the work of the reasoning intelligence and does much more, but with a greater power and in a different fashion. It is then itself taken up into a higher range of the power of knowledge and in that too nothing is lost, but all farther heightened, enlarged in scope, transformed in power of action.

The ordinary language of the intellect is not sufficient to describe this action, for the same words have to be used, indicating a certain correspondence, but actually to connote inadequately a different thing. Thus the supermind uses a certain sense action, employing but not limited by the physical organs, a thing which is in its nature a form consciousness and a contact consciousness, but the mental idea and experience of sense can give no conception of the essential and characteristic action of this supramentalised sense consciousness. Thought too in the supramental action is a different thing from the thought of the mental intelligence. The supramental thinking is felt at its basis as a conscious contact or union or identity of the substance of being of the knower with the substance of being of the thing known and its figure of thought as the power of awareness of the self revealing through the meeting or the oneness, because carrying in itself, a certain knowledge form of the object's content, action, significance. Therefore observation, memory, judgment too mean each a different thing in the supermind from what it is in the process of the mental intelligence.

The supramental reason observes all that the intelligence observes—and much more; it makes, that is to say, the thing to be known the field of a perceptual action, in a certain way objective, that causes to emerge its nature, character, quality, action. But this is not that artificial objectivity by which the reason in its observation tries to extrude the element of personal or subjective error. The supermind sees everything in the self and its observation must therefore be subjectively objective and much nearer to, though not the same as the observation of our own internal movements regarded as an object of knowledge. It is not in the separatively personal self or by its power that it sees and therefore it has not to be on guard against the element of personal error: that interferes only while a mental substratum or environing atmosphere yet remains and can still throw in its influence or while the supermind is still acting by descent into the mind to change it. And the supramental method with error is to eliminate it, not by any other device, but by an increasing spontaneity of the supramental discrimination and a constant heightening of its own energy. The consciousness of supermind is a cosmic consciousness and it is in this self of universal consciousness, in which the individual knower lives and with which he is more or less closely united, that it holds before him the object of knowledge.

The knower is in his observation a witness and this relation would seem to imply an otherness and difference, but the point is that it is not an entirely separative difference and does not bring an excluding idea of the thing observed as completely not self, as in the mental seeing of an external object. There is always a basic feeling of oneness with the thing known, for without this oneness there can be no supramental knowledge. The knower carrying the object in his universalised self of consciousness as a thing held before his station of witness vision includes it in his own wider being. The supramental observation is of things with which we are one in the being and consciousness and are capable of knowing them even as we know ourselves by the force of that oneness: the act of observation is a movement towards bringing out the latent knowledge.

There is, then, first a fundamental unity of consciousness that is greater or less in its power, more or less completely and immediately revelatory of its contents of knowledge according to our progress and elevation and intensity of living, feeling and seeing in the supramental ranges. There is set up between the knower and the object of knowledge, as a result of this fundamental unity, a stream or bridge of conscious connection—one is obliged to use images, however inadequate—and as a consequence a contact or active union enabling one to see, feel, sense supramentally what is to be known in the object or about it. Sometimes this stream or bridge of connection is not sensibly felt at the moment, only the results of the contact are noted, but it is always really there and an after memory can always make us aware that it was really all the time present: as we grow in supramentality, it becomes an abiding factor. The necessity of this stream or this bridge of connection ceases when the fundamental oneness becomes a complete active oneness. This process is the basis of what Patanjali calls *saṁyama*, a concentration, directing or dwelling of the consciousness, by which, he says, one can become aware of all that is in the object. But the necessity of concentration becomes slight or nil when the active oneness grows; the luminous consciousness of the object and its contents becomes more spontaneous, normal, facile.

There are three possible movements of this kind of supramental observation. First, the knower may project himself in consciousness on the object, feel his cognition in contact or enveloping or penetrating it and there, as it were in the object itself, become aware of what he has to know. Or he may by the contact become aware of that which is in it or belongs to it, as for example the thought or feeling of another, coming from it and entering into himself where he stands in his station of the witness. Or he may simply know in himself by a sort of supramental cognition in his own witness station without any such projection or entrance. The starting-point and apparent basis of the observation may be the presence of the object to the physical or other senses, but to the supermind this is not indispensable. It may be instead an inner image or simply the idea of the object. The simple will to know may bring to the supramental consciousness the needed knowledge—or, it may be, the will to be known or communicate itself of the object of knowledge.

The elaborate process of analytical observation and synthetical construction adopted by the logical intelligence is not the method of the supermind and yet there is a corresponding action. The supermind distinguishes by a direct seeing and without any mental process of taking to pieces the particularities of the thing, form, energy, action, quality, mind, soul that it has in view, and it sees too with an equal directness and without any process of construction the significant totality of which these particularities are the incidents. It sees also the essentiality, the Swabhava, of the thing in itself of which the totality and the particularities are the manifestation. And again it sees, whether apart from or through the essentiality or swabhava, the one self, the one existence, consciousness, power, force of which it is the basic expression.

It may be observing at the time only the particularities, but the whole is implied, and *vice versa*,—as for an example, the total state of mind out of which a thought or a feeling arises,—and the cognition may start from one or the other and proceed at once by immediate suggestion to the implied knowledge. The essentiality is similarly implied in the whole and in each or all of the particulars and there may be the same rapid or immediate alternative or alternate process. The logic of the supermind is different from that of the mind: it sees always the self as what is, the essentiality of the thing as a fundamental expression of the being and power of the self, and the whole and particulars as a consequent manifestation of this power and its active expression. In the fullness of the supramental consciousness and cognition this is the constant order. All perception of unity, similarity, difference, kind, uniqueness arrived at by the supramental reason is consonant with and depends on this order.

This observing action of supermind applies to all things. Its view of physical objects is not and cannot be only a surface or outward view, even when concentrated on the externals. It sees the form, action, properties, but it is aware at the same time of the qualities or energies, *guṇa*, *śakti*, of which the form is a translation, and it sees them not as an inference or deduction from the form or action, but feels and sees them directly in the being of the object and quite as vividly,—one might say, with a subtle concreteness and fine substantiality,—as the form or sensible action. It is aware too of the consciousness that manifests itself in quality, energy, form. It can feel, know, observe, see forces, tendencies, impulsions, things abstract to us quite as directly and vividly as the things we now call visible and sensible. It observes in just the same way persons and beings. It can take as its starting-point or first indication the speech, action, outward signs, but it is not limited by or dependent on them. It can know and feel and observe the very self and consciousness of another, can either proceed to that directly through the sign or can in its more powerful action begin with it and at once, instead of seeking to know the inner being through the evidence of the outer expression, understand rather all the outer expression in the light of the inner being. Even so, completely, the supramental being knows his own inner being and nature. The supermind can too act with equal power and observe with direct experience what is hidden behind the physical order; it can move in other planes than the material universe. It knows the self and reality of things by identity, by experience of oneness or contact of oneness and a vision, a seeing and realising ideation and knowledge dependent on or derived from these things, and its thought presentation of the truths of the spirit is an expression of this kind of sight and experience.

The supramental memory is different from the mental, not a storing up of past knowledge and experience, but an abiding presence of knowledge that can be brought forward or, more characteristically, offers itself, when it is needed: it is not dependent on attention or on conscious reception, for the things of the past not known actually or not observed can be called up from latency by an action which is yet essentially a remembrance. Especially on a certain level all knowledge presents itself as a remembering, because all is latent or inherent in the self of supermind. The future like the past presents itself to knowledge in the supermind as a memory of the preknown. The imagination transformed in the supermind acts on one side as a power of true image and symbol, always an image or index of some value or significance or other truth of being, on the other as an inspiration or interpretative seeing of possibilities and potentialities not less true than actual or realised things. These are put in their place either by an attendant intuitive or interpretative judgment or by one inherent in the vision of the image, symbol or potentiality, or by a supereminent revelation of that which is behind the image or symbol or which determines the potential and the actual and their relations and, it may be, overrides and overpasses them, imposing ultimate truths and supreme certitudes.

The supramental judgment acts inseparably from the supramental observation or memory, inherent in it as a direct seeing or cognition of values, significances, antecedents, consequences, relations, etc.; or it supervenes on the observation as a luminous disclosing idea or suggestion; or it may go before, independent of any observation, and then the object called up and observed confirms visibly the truth of the idea. But in each case it is sufficient in itself for its own purpose, is its own evidence and does not really depend for its truth on any aid or confirmation. There is a logic of the supramental reason, but its function is not to test or scrutinise, to support and prove or to detect and eliminate error. Its function is simply to link knowledge with knowledge, to discover and utilise harmonies and arrangement and relations, to organise the movement of the supramental knowledge. This it does not by any formal rule or construction of inferences but by a direct, living and immediate seeing and placing of connection and relation. All thought in the supermind is in the nature of intuition, inspiration or revelation and all deficiency of knowledge is to be supplied by a farther action of these powers; error is prevented by the action of a spontaneous and luminous discrimination; the movement is always from knowledge to knowledge. It is not rational in our sense but suprarational,—it does sovereignly what is sought to be done stumblingly and imperfectly by the mental reason.

The ranges of knowledge above the supramental reason, taking it up and exceeding it, cannot well be described, nor is it necessary here to make the endeavour. It is sufficient to say that the process here is more sufficient, intense and large in light, imperative, instantaneous, the scope of the active knowledge larger, the way nearer to the knowledge by identity, the thought more packed with the luminous substance of self-awareness and all-vision and more evidently independent of any other inferior support or assistance.

These characteristics, it must be remembered, do not fully apply even to the strongest action of the intuitive mentality, but are there seen only in their first glimpses. Nor can they be entirely or unmixedly evident so long as supramentality is only forming with an undercurrent, a mixture or an environment of mental action. It is only when mentality is overpassed and drops away into a passive silence that there can be the full disclosure and the sovereign and integral action of the supramental gnosis.

# THE SUPRAMENTAL SENSE

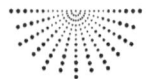

ALL THE instruments, all the activities of the mind have their corresponding powers in the action of the supramental energy and are there exalted and transfigured, but have there a reverse order of priority and necessary importance. As there is a supramental thought and essential consciousness, so too there is a supramental sense. Sense is fundamentally not the action of certain physical organs, but the contact of consciousness with its objects, *saṁjñāna*.

When the consciousness of the being is withdrawn wholly into itself, it is aware only of itself, of its own being, its own consciousness, its own delight of existence, its own concentrated force of being, and of these things not in their forms but in their essence. When it comes out of this self-immersion, it becomes aware of or it releases or develops out of its self-immersion its activities and forms of being, of consciousness, of delight and force. Then too, on the supramental plane, its primary awareness still remains of a kind native to and entirely characteristic of the self-awareness of the spirit, the self-knowledge of the one and infinite; it is a knowledge that knows all its objects, forms and activities comprehensively by being aware of them in its own infinite self, intimately by being aware in them as their self, absolutely by being aware of them as one in self with its own being. All its other ways of knowledge are projected from this knowledge by identity, are parts or movements of it, or at the lowest depend on it for their truth and light, are touched and supported by it even in their own separate way of action and refer back to it overtly or implicitly as their authority and origin.

The activity which is nearest to this essential knowledge by identity is the large embracing consciousness, especially characteristic of the supramental energy, which takes into itself all truth and idea and object of knowledge and sees them at once in their essence, totality and parts or aspects,—*vijñāna*. Its movement is a total seeing and seizing; it is a comprehension and possession in the self of knowledge; and it holds the object of consciousness as a part of the self or one with it, the unity being spontaneously and directly realised in the act of knowledge. Another supramental activity puts the knowledge by identity more into the background and stresses more the objectivity of the thing known. Its characteristic movement, descending into the mind, becomes the source of the peculiar nature of our mental knowledge, intelligence, *prajñāna*. In the mind the action of intelligence involves, at the outset, separation and otherness between the knower, knowledge and the known; but in the supermind its movement still takes place in the infinite identity or at least in the cosmic oneness. Only, the self of knowledge indulges the delight of putting the object of consciousness away from the more immediate nearness of the original and eternal unity, but always in itself, and of knowing it again in another way so as to establish with it a variety of relations of interaction which are so many minor chords in the harmony of the play of the consciousness. The movement of this supramental intelligence, *prajñāna*, becomes a subordinate, a tertiary action of the supramental for the fullness of which thought and word are needed. The primary action, because it is of the nature of knowledge by identity or of a comprehensive seizing in the consciousness, is complete in itself and has no need of these means of formulation. The supramental intelligence is of the nature of a truth seeing, truth hearing and truth remembering and, though capable of being sufficient to itself in a certain way, still feels itself more richly fulfilled by the thought and word that give it a body of expression.

Finally, a fourth action of the supramental consciousness completes the various possibilities of the supramental knowledge. This still farther accentuates the objectivity of the thing known, puts it away from the station of experiencing consciousness and again brings it to nearness by a uniting contact effected either in a direct nearness, touch, union or less closely across the bridge or through the connecting stream of consciousness of which there has already been mention. It is a contacting of existence, presences, things, forms, forces, activities, but a contacting of them in the stuff of the supramental being and energy, not in the divisions of matter and through the physical instruments, that creates the supramental sense, *saṁjñāna*.

It is a little difficult to make the nature of the supramental sense understood to a mentality not yet familiar with it by enlarged experience, because our idea of sense action is governed by the limiting experience of the physical mind and we suppose that the fundamental thing in it is the impression made by an external object on the physical organ of sight, hearing, smell, touch, taste, and that the business of the mind, the present central organ of our consciousness, is only to receive the physical impression and its nervous translation and so become intelligently conscious of the object. In order to understand the supramental change we have to realise first that the mind is the only real sense even in the physical process: its dependence on the physical impressions is the result of the conditions of the material evolution, but not a thing fundamental and indispensable. Mind is capable of a sight that is independent of the physical eye, a hearing that is independent of the physical ear, and so with the action of all the other senses. It is capable too of an awareness, operating by what appears to us as mental impressions, of things not conveyed or even suggested by the agency of the physical organs,—an opening to relations, happenings, forms even and the action of forces to which the physical organs could not have borne evidence. Then, becoming aware of these rarer powers, we speak of the mind as a sixth sense; but in fact it is the only true sense organ and the rest are no more than its outer conveniences and secondary instruments, although by its dependence on them they have become its limitations and its too imperative and exclusive conveyors. Again we have to realise—and this is more difficult to admit for our normal ideas in the matter—that the mind itself is only the characteristic instrument of sense, but the thing itself, sense in its purity, *saṁjñāna*, exists behind and beyond the mind it uses and is a movement of the self, a direct and original activity of the infinite power of its consciousness.

The pure action of sense is a spiritual action and pure sense is itself a power of the spirit.

The spiritual sense is capable of knowing in its own characteristic way, which is other than that of supramental thought or of the intelligence or spiritual comprehension, *vijñāna*, or knowledge by identity, all things whatsoever, things material and what is to us immaterial, all forms and that which is formless. For all is spiritual substance of being, substance of consciousness and force, substance of delight; and the spiritual sense, pure *saṁjñāna*, is the conscious being's contactual, substantial awareness of its own extended substance of self and in it of all that is of the infinite or universal substance. It is possible for us not only to know by conscious identity, by a spiritual comprehension of self, of principles and aspects, force, play and action, by a direct spiritual, supramental and intuitive thought knowledge, by the heart's spiritually and supramentally illumined feeling, love, delight, but also to have in a very literal significance the sense—sense-knowledge or sensation—of the spirit, the self, the Divine, the Infinite. The state described by the Upanishad in which one sees, hears, feels, touches, senses in every way the Brahman and the Brahman only, for all things have become to the consciousness only that and have no other, separate or independent existence, is not a mere figure of speech, but the exact description of the fundamental action of the pure sense, the spiritual object of the pure *saṁjñāna*. And in this original action,—to our experience a transfigured, glorified, infinitely blissful action of the sense, a direct feeling out inward, around, everywhere of the self to embrace and touch and be sensible of all that is in its universal being,—we can become aware in a most moving and delightful way of the Infinite and of all that is in it, cognizant, by intimate contact of our being with all being, of whatever is in the universe.

The action of the supramental sense is founded on this true truth of sense; it is an organisation of this pure, spiritual, infinite, absolute *saṁjñāna*. The supermind acting through sense feels all as God and in God, all as the manifest touch, sight, hearing, taste, perfume, all as the felt, seen, directly experienced substance and power and energy and movement, play, penetration, vibration, form, nearness, pressure, substantial interchange of the Infinite. Nothing exists independently to its sense, but all is felt as one being and movement and each thing as indivisible from the rest and as having in it all the Infinite, all the Divine. This supramental sense has the direct feeling and experience, not only of forms, but of forces and of the energy and the quality in things and of a divine substance and presence which is within them and round them and into which they open and expand themselves in their secret subtle self and elements, extending themselves in oneness into the illimitable. Nothing to the supramental sense is really finite: it is founded on a feeling of all in each and of each in all: its sense definition, although more precise and complete than the mental, creates no walls of limitation; it is an oceanic and ethereal sense in which all particular sense knowledge and sensation is a wave or movement or spray or drop that is yet a concentration of the whole ocean and inseparable from the ocean. Its action is a result of the extension and vibration of being and consciousness in a supra-ethereal ether of light, ether of power, ether of bliss, the Ananda Akasha of the Upanishads, which is the matrix and continent of the universal expression of the Self,—here in body and mind experienced only in limited extensions and vibrations,—and the medium of its true experience. This sense even at its lowest power is luminous with a revealing light that carries in it the secret of the thing it experiences and can therefore be a starting-point and basis of all the rest of the supramental knowledge,—the supramental thought, spiritual intelligence and comprehension, conscious identity,—and on its highest plane or at its fullest intensity of action it opens into or contains and at once liberates these things. It is strong with a luminous power that carries in it the force of self-realisation and an intense or infinite effectiveness, and this sense-experience can therefore be the starting-point of impulsion for a creative or fulfilling action of the spiritual and supramental will and knowledge. It is rapturous with a powerful and luminous delight that makes of it, makes of all sense and sensation a key to or a vessel of the divine and infinite Ananda.

The supramental sense can act in its own power and is independent of the body and the physical life and outer mind and it is above too the inner mind and its experiences. It can be aware of all things in whatever world, on whatever plane, in whatever formation of universal consciousness. It can be aware of the things of the material universe even in the trance of samadhi, aware of them as they are or appear to the physical sense, even as it is of other states of experience, of the pure vital, the mental, the psychical, the supramental presentation of things. It can in the waking state of the physical consciousness present to us the things concealed from the limited receptivity or beyond the range of the physical organs, distant forms, scenes and happenings, things that have passed out of physical existence or that are not yet in physical existence, scenes, forms, happenings, symbols of the vital, psychical, mental, supramental, spiritual worlds and all these in their real or significant truth as well as their appearance. It can use all the other states of sense consciousness and their appropriate senses and organs adding to them what they have not, setting right their errors and supplying their deficiencies: for it is the source of the others and they are only inferior derivations from this higher sense, this true and illimitable *saṁjñāna*.

The lifting of the level of consciousness from the mind to the supermind and the consequent transformation of the being from the state of the mental to that of the supramental Purusha must bring with it to be complete a transformation of all the parts of the nature and all its activities. The whole mind is not merely made into a passive channel of the supramental activities, a channel of their downflow into the life and body and of their outflow or communication with the outward world, the material existence,—that is only the first stage of the process,—but is itself supramentalised along with all its instruments. There is accordingly a change, a profound transformation in the physical sense, a supramentalising of the physical sight, hearing, touch, etc., that creates or reveals to us a quite different view, not merely of life and its meaning, but even of the material world and all its forms and aspects. The supermind uses the physical organs and confirms their way of action, but it develops behind them the inner and deeper senses which see what are hidden from the physical organs and farther transforms the new sight, hearing, etc. thus created by casting it into its own mould and way of sensing. The change is one that takes nothing from the physical truth of the object, but adds to it its supraphysical truth and takes away by the removal of the physical limitation the element of falsehood in the material way of experience.

The supramentalising of the physical sense brings with it a result similar in this field to that which we experience in the transmutation of the thought and consciousness. As soon as the sight, for example, becomes altered under the influence of the supramental seeing, the eye gets a new and transfigured vision of things and of the world around us. Its sight acquires an extraordinary totality and an immediate and embracing precision in which the whole and every detail stand out at once in the complete harmony and vividness of the significance meant by Nature in the object and its realisation of the idea in form, executed in a triumph of substantial being. It is as if the eye of the poet and artist had replaced the vague or trivial unseeing normal vision, but singularly spiritualised and glorified,—as if indeed it were the sight of the supreme divine Poet and Artist in which we were participating and there were given to us the full seeing of his truth and intention in his design of the universe and of each thing in the universe. There is an unlimited intensity which makes all that is seen a revelation of the glory of quality and idea and form and colour. The physical eye seems then to carry in itself a spirit and a consciousness which sees not only the physical aspect of the object but the soul of quality in it, the vibration of energy, the light and force and spiritual substance of which it is made. Thus there comes through the physical sense to the total sense consciousness within and behind the vision a revelation of the soul of the thing seen and of the universal spirit that is expressing itself in this objective form of its own conscious being.

There is at the same time a subtle change which makes the sight see in a sort of fourth dimension, the character of which is a certain internality, the seeing not only of the superficies and the outward form but of that which informs it and subtly extends around it. The material object becomes to this sight something different from what we now see, not a separate object on the background or in the environment of the rest of Nature, but an indivisible part and even in a subtle way an expression of the unity of all that we see. And this unity that we see becomes not only to the subtler consciousness but to the mere sense, to the illumined physical sight itself, that of the identity of the Eternal, the unity of the Brahman. For to the supramentalised seeing the material world and space and material objects cease to be material in the sense in which we now on the strength of the sole evidence of our limited physical organs and of the physical consciousness that looks through them receive as our gross perception and understand as our conception of matter. It and they appear and are seen as spirit itself in a form of itself and a conscious extension. The whole is a unity—the oneness unaffected by any multitudinousness of objects and details—held in and by the consciousness in a spiritual space and all substance there is conscious substance. This change and this totality of the way of seeing comes from the exceeding of the limitations of our present physical sense, because the power of the subtle or psychical eye has been infused into the physical and there has again been infused into this psycho-physical power of vision the spiritual sight, the pure sense, the supramental *saṁjñāna*.

All the other senses undergo a similar transformation. All that the ear listens to, reveals the totality of its sound body and sound significance and all the tones of its vibration and reveals also to the single and complete hearing the quality, the rhythmic energy, the soul of the sound and its expression of the one universal spirit. There is the same internality, the going of the sense into the depths of the sound and the finding there of that which informs it and extends it into unity with the harmony of all sound and no less with the harmony of all silence, so that the ear is always listening to the infinite in its heard expression and the voice of its silence. All sounds become to the supramentalised ear the voice of the Divine, himself born into sound, and a rhythm of the concord of the universal symphony. And there is too the same completeness, vividness, intensity, the revelation of the self of the thing heard and the spiritual satisfaction of the self in hearing. The supramentalised touch also contacts or receives the touch of the Divine in all things and knows all things as the Divine through the conscious self in the contact: and there is too the same totality, intensity, revelation of all that is in and behind the touch to the experiencing consciousness. There comes a similar transformation of the other senses.

There is at the same time an opening of new powers in all the senses, an extension of range, a stretching out of the physical consciousness to an undreamed capacity. The supramental transformation extends too the physical consciousness far beyond the limits of the body and enables it to receive with a perfect concreteness the physical contact of things at a distance. And the physical organs become capable of serving as channels for the psychic and other senses so that we can see with the physical waking eye what is ordinarily revealed only in the abnormal states and to the psychical vision, hearing or other sense knowledge. It is the spirit or the inner soul that sees and senses, but the body and its powers are themselves spiritualised and share directly in the experience. The entire material sensation is supramentalised and it becomes aware, directly and with a physical participation and, finally, a unity with the subtler instrumentation, of forces and movements and the physical, vital, emotional, mental vibrations of things and beings and feels them all not only spiritually or mentally but physically in the self and as movements of the one self in these many bodies. The wall that the limitations of the body and its senses have built around us is abolished even in the body and the senses and there is in its place the free communication of the eternal oneness. All sense and sensation becomes full of the divine light, the divine power and intensity of experience, a divine joy, the delight of the Brahman. And even that which is now to us discordant and jars on the senses takes its place in the universal concord of the universal movement, reveals its *rasa*, meaning, design and, by delight in its intention in the divine consciousness and its manifestation of its law and dharma, its harmony with the total self, its place in the manifestation of the divine being, becomes beautiful and happy to the soul experience. All sensation becomes Ananda.

The embodied mind in us is ordinarily aware only through the physical organs and only of their objects and of subjective experiences which seem to start from the physical experience and to take them alone, however remotely, for their foundation and mould of construction. All the rest, all that is not consistent with or part of or verified by the physical data, seems to it rather imagination than reality and it is only in abnormal states that it opens to other kinds of conscious experience. But in fact there are immense ranges behind of which we could be aware if we opened the doors of our inner being. These ranges are there already in action and known to a subliminal self in us, and much even of our surface consciousness is directly projected from them and without our knowing it influences our subjective experience of things. There is a range of independent vital or pranic experiences behind, subliminal to and other than the surface action of the vitalised physical consciousness. And when this opens itself or acts in any way, there are made manifest to the waking mind the phenomena of a vital consciousness, a vital intuition, a vital sense not dependent on the body and its instruments, although it may use them as a secondary medium and a recorder. It is possible to open completely this range and, when we do so, we find that its operation is that of the conscious life force individualised in us contacting the universal life force and its operations in things, happenings and persons. The mind becomes aware of the life consciousness in all things, responds to it through our life consciousness with an immediate directness not limited by the ordinary communication through the body and its organs, records its intuitions, becomes capable of experiencing existence as a translation of the universal Life or Prana. The field of which the vital consciousness and the vital sense are primarily aware is not that of forms but, directly, that of forces: its world is a world of the play of energies, and form and event are sensed only secondarily as a result and embodiment of the energies. The mind working through the physical senses can only construct a view and knowledge of this nature as an idea in the intelligence, but it cannot go beyond the physical translation of the energies, and it has therefore no real or direct experience of the true nature of life, no actual realisation of the life force and the life spirit. It is by opening this other level or depth of experience within and by admission to the vital consciousness and vital sense that the mind can get the true and direct experience. Still, even then, so long as it is on the mental level, the experience is limited by the vital terms and their mental renderings and there is an obscurity even in this greatened sense and knowledge. The supramental transformation supravitalises the vital, reveals it as a dynamics of the spirit, makes a complete opening and a true revelation of all the spiritual reality behind and within the life force and the life spirit and of all its spiritual as well as its mental and purely vital truth and significance.

The supermind in its descent into the physical being awakens, if not already wakened by previous yogic sadhana, the consciousness—veiled or obscure in most of us—which supports and forms there the vitals heath, the *prāṇakoṣa*. When this is awakened, we no longer live in the physical body alone, but also in a vital body which penetrates and envelops the physical and is sensitive to impacts of another kind, to the play of the vital forces around us and coming in on us from the universe or from particular persons or group lives or from things or else from the vital planes and worlds which are behind the material universe. These impacts we feel even now in their result and in certain touches and affectations, but not at all or very little in their source and their coming. An awakened consciousness in the pranic body immediately feels them, is aware of a pervading vital force other than the physical energy, and can draw upon it to increase the vital strength and support the physical energies, can deal directly with the phenomena and causes of health and disease by means of this vital influx or by directing pranic currents, can be aware of the vital and the vital-emotional atmosphere of others and deal with its interchanges, along with a host of other phenomena which are unfelt by or obscure to our outward consciousness but here become conscient and sensible. It is acutely aware of the life soul and life body in ourself and others. The supermind takes up this vital consciousness and vital sense, puts it on its right foundation and transforms it by revealing the life-force here as the very power of the spirit dynamised for a near and direct operation on and through subtle and gross matter and for formation and action in the material universe.

The first result is that the limitations of our individual life being break down and we live no longer with a personal life force, or not with that ordinarily, but in and by the universal life energy. It is all the universal Prana that comes consciently streaming into and through us, keeps up there a dynamic constant eddy, an unseparated centre of its power, a vibrant station of storage and communication, constantly fills it with its forces and pours them out in activity upon the world around us. This life energy, again, is felt by us not merely as a vital ocean and its streams, but as the vital way and form and body and outpouring of a conscious universal Shakti, and that conscient Shakti reveals itself as the Chit Shakti of the Divine, the Energy of the transcendent and universal Self and Purusha of which—or rather of whom—our universalised individuality becomes an instrument and channel. As a result we feel ourselves one in life with all others and one with the life of all Nature and of all things in the universe. There is a free and conscious communication of the vital energy working in us with the same energy working in others. We are aware of their life as of our own or, at the least, of the touch and pressure and communicated movements of our life being on them and theirs upon us. The vital sense in us becomes powerful, intense, capable of bearing all the small or large, minute or immense vibrations of this life world on all its planes physical and supraphysical, vital and supravital, thrills with all its movement and Ananda and is aware of and open to all forces. The supermind takes possession of all this great range of experience, and makes it all luminous, harmonious, experienced not obscurely and fragmentarily and subject to the limitations and errors of its handling by the mental ignorance, but revealed, it and each movement of it, in its truth and totality of power and delight, and directs the great and now hardly limitable powers and capacities of the life dynamis on all its ranges according to the simple and yet complex, the sheer and spontaneous and yet unfalteringly intricate will of the Divine in our life. It makes the vital sense a perfect means of the knowledge of the life forces around us, as the physical of the forms and sensations of the physical universe, and a perfect channel too of the reactions of the active life force through us working as an instrument of self-manifestation.

The phenomena of this vital consciousness and sense, this direct sensation and perception of and response to the play of subtler forces than the physical, are often included without distinction under the head of psychical phenomena. In a certain sense it is an awakening of the psyche, the inner soul now hidden, clogged wholly or partially covered up by the superficial activity of the physical mind and senses that brings to the surface the submerged or subliminal inner vital consciousness and also an inner or subliminal mental consciousness and sense capable of perceiving and experiencing directly, not only the life forces and their play and results and phenomena, but the mental and psychical worlds and all they contain and the mental activities, vibrations, phenomena, forms, images of this world also and of establishing a direct communication between mind and mind without the aid of the physical organs and the limitations they impose on our consciousness. There are however two different kinds of action of these inner ranges of the consciousness. The first is a more outer and confused activity of the awakening subliminal mind and life which is clogged with and subject to the grosser desires and illusions of the mind and vital being and vitiated in spite of its wider range of experience and powers and capacities by an enormous mass of error and deformations of the will and knowledge, full of false suggestions and images, false and distorted intuitions and inspirations and impulses, the latter often even depraved and perverse, and vitiated too by the interference of the physical mind and its obscurities. This is an inferior activity to which clairvoyants, psychists, spiritists, occultists, seekers of powers and siddhis are very liable and to which all the warnings against the dangers and errors of this kind of seeking are more especially applicable. The seeker of spiritual perfection has to pass as quickly as possible, if he cannot altogether avoid, this zone of danger, and the safe rule here is to be attached to none of these things, but to make spiritual progress one's sole real objective and to put no sure confidence in other things until the mind and life soul are purified and the light of the spirit and supermind or at least of the spiritually illumined mind and soul are shed on these inner ranges of experience. For when the mind is tranquillised and purified and the pure psyche liberated from the insistence of the desire soul, these experiences are free from any serious danger,—except indeed that of limitation and a certain element of error which cannot be entirely eliminated so long as the soul experiences and acts on the mental level. For there is then a pure action of the true psychical consciousness and its powers, a reception of psychical experience pure in itself of the worse deformations, although subject to the limitations of the representing mind, and capable of a high spiritualisation and light. The complete power and truth, however, can only come by the opening of the supermind and the supramentalising of the mental and psychical experience.

The range of the psychic consciousness and its experiences is almost illimitable and the variety and complexity of its phenomena almost infinite. Only some of the broad lines and main features can be noted here. The first and most prominent is the activity of the psychic senses of which the sight is the most developed ordinarily and the first to manifest itself with any largeness when the veil of the absorption in the surface consciousness which prevents the inner vision is broken. But all the physical senses have their corresponding powers in the psychical being, there is a psychical hearing, touch, smell, taste: indeed the physical senses are themselves in reality only a projection of the inner sense into a limited and externalised operation in and through and upon the phenomena of gross matter. The psychical sight receives characteristically the images that are formed in the subtle matter of the mental or psychical ether, *cittākāśa*. These may be transcriptions there or impresses of physical things, persons, scenes, happenings, whatever is, was or will be or may be in the physical universe. These images are very variously seen and under all kinds of conditions; in samadhi or in the waking state, and in the latter with the bodily eyes closed or open, projected on or into a physical object or medium or seen as if materialised in the physical atmosphere or only in a psychical ether revealing itself through this grosser physical atmosphere; seen through the physical eyes themselves as a secondary instrument and as if under the conditions of the physical vision or by the psychical vision alone and independently of the relations of our ordinary sight to space. The real agent is always the psychical sight and the power indicates that the consciousness is more or less awake, intermittently or normally and more or less perfectly, in the psychical body. It is possible to see in this way the transcriptions or impressions of things at any distance beyond the range of the physical vision or the images of the past or the future.

Besides these transcriptions or impresses the psychical vision receives thought images and other forms created by constant activity of consciousness in ourselves or in other human beings, and these may be according to the character of the activity images of truth or falsehood or else mixed things, partly true, partly false, and may be too either mere shells and representations or images inspired with a temporary life and consciousness and, it may be, carrying in them in one way or another some kind of beneficent or maleficent action or some willed or unwilled effectiveness on our minds or vital being or through them even on the body. These transcriptions, impresses, thought images, life images, projections of the consciousness may also be representations or creations not of the physical world, but of vital, psychic or mental worlds beyond us, seen in our own minds or projected from other than human beings. And as there is this psychical vision of which some of the more external and ordinary manifestations are well enough known by the name of clairvoyance, so there is a psychical hearing and psychical touch, taste, smell—clairaudience, clairsentience are the more external manifestations, —with precisely the same range each in its own kind, the same fields and manner and conditions and varieties of their phenomena.

These and other phenomena create an indirect, a representative range of psychical experience; but the psychical sense has also the power of putting us in a more direct communication with earthly or supraterrestrial beings through their psychical selves or their psychical bodies or even with things, for things also have a psychical reality and souls or presences supporting them which can communicate with our psychical consciousness. The most notable of these more powerful but rarer phenomena are those which attend the power of exteriorisation of our consciousness for various kinds of action otherwise and elsewhere than in the physical body, communication in the psychical body or some emanation or reproduction of it, oftenest, though by no means necessarily, during sleep or trance and the setting up of relations or communication by various means with the denizens of another plane of existence.

For there is a continuous scale of the planes of consciousness, beginning with the psychical and other belts attached to and dependent on the earth plane and proceeding through the true independent vital and psychical worlds to the worlds of the gods and the highest supramental and spiritual planes of existence. And these are in fact always acting upon our subliminal selves unknown to our waking mind and with considerable effect on our life and nature. The physical mind is only a little part of us and there is a much more considerable range of our being in which the presence, influence and powers of the other planes are active upon us and help to shape our external being and its activities. The awakening of the psychical consciousness enables us to become aware of these powers, presences and influences in and around us; and while in the impure or yet ignorant and imperfect mind this unveiled contact has its dangers, it enables us too, if rightly used and directed, to be no longer their subject but their master and to come into conscious and self-controlled possession of the inner secrets of our nature. The psychical consciousness reveals this interaction between the inner and the outer planes, this world and others, partly by an awareness, which may be very constant, vast and vivid, of their impacts, suggestions, communications to our inner thought and conscious being and a capacity of reaction upon them there, partly also through many kinds of symbolic, transcriptive or representative images presented to the different psychical senses. But also there is the possibility of a more direct, concretely sensible, almost material, sometimes actively material communication—a complete though temporary physical materialisation seems to be possible—with the powers, forces and beings of other worlds and planes. There may even be a complete breaking of the limits of the physical consciousness and the material existence.

The awakening of the psychical consciousness liberates in us the direct use of the mind as a sixth sense, and this power may be made constant and normal. The physical consciousness can only communicate with the minds of others or know the happenings of the world around us through external means and signs and indications, and it has beyond this limited action only a vague and haphazard use of the mind's more direct capacities, a poor range of occasional presentiments, intuitions and messages. Our minds are indeed constantly acting and acted upon by the minds of others through hidden currents of which we are not aware, but we have no knowledge or control of these agencies. The psychical consciousness, as it develops, makes us aware of the great mass of thoughts, feelings, suggestions, will impacts, influences of all kinds that we are receiving from others or sending to others or imbibing from and throwing into the general mind atmosphere around us. As it evolves in power, precision and clearness, we are able to trace these to their source or feel immediately their origin and transit to us and direct consciously and with an intelligent will our own messages. It becomes possible to be aware, more or less accurately and discerningly, of the activities of minds whether near to us physically or at a distance, to understand, feel or identify ourselves with their temperament, character, thoughts, feelings, reactions, whether by a psychic sense or a direct mental perception or by a very sensible and often intensely concrete reception of them into our mind or on its recording surface. At the same time we can consciously make at least the inner selves and, if they are sufficiently sensitive, the surface minds of others aware of our own inner mental or psychic self and plastic to its thoughts, suggestions, influences or even cast it or its active image in influence into their subjective, even into their vital and physical being to work there as a helping or moulding or dominating power and presence.

All these powers of the psychic consciousness need have and often have no more than a mental utility and significance, but it can also be used with a spiritual sense and light and intention in it and for a spiritual purpose. This can be done by a spiritual meaning and use in our psychical interchange with others, and it is largely by a psycho-spiritual interchange of this kind that a master in Yoga helps his disciple. The knowledge of our inner subliminal and psychic nature, of the powers and presences and influences there and the capacity of communication with other planes and their powers and beings can also be used for a higher than any mental or mundane object, for the possession and mastering of our whole nature and the overpassing of the intermediate planes on the way to the supreme spiritual heights of being. But the most direct spiritual use of the psychic consciousness is to make it an instrument of contact, communication and union with the Divine. A world of psycho-spiritual symbols is readily opened up, illuminating and potent and living forms and instruments, which can be made a revelation of spiritual significances, a support for our spiritual growth and the evolution of spiritual capacity and experience, a means towards spiritual power, knowledge or Ananda. The mantra is one of these psycho-spiritual means, at once a symbol, an instrument and a sound body for the divine manifestation, and of the same kind are the images of the Godhead and of its personalities or powers used in meditation or for adoration in Yoga. The great forms or bodies of the Divine are revealed through which he manifests his living presence to us and we can more easily by their means intimately know, adore and give ourselves to him and enter into the different lokas, worlds of his habitation and presence, where we can live in the light of his being. His word, command, Adesha, presence, touch, guidance can come to us through our spiritualised psychic consciousness and, as a subtly concrete means of transmission from the spirit, it can give us a close communication and nearness to him through all our psychic senses. These and many more are the spiritual uses of the psychic consciousness and sense and, although capable of limitation and deformation,—for all secondary instruments can be also by our mental capacity of exclusive self-limitation means of a partial but at the same time hindrances to a more integral realisation,—they are of the greatest utility on the road to the spiritual perfection and afterwards, liberated from the limitation of our minds, transformed and supramentalised, an element of rich detail in the spiritual Ananda.

As the physical and vital, the psychical consciousness and sense also are capable of a supramental transformation and receive by it their own integral fullness and significance. The supermind lays hold on the psychical being, descends into it, changes it into the mould of its own nature and uplifts it to be a part of the supramental action and state, the supra-psychic being of the Vijnana Purusha. The first result of this change is to base the phenomena of the psychical consciousness on their true foundation by bringing into it the permanent sense, the complete realisation, the secure possession of the oneness of our mind and soul with the minds and souls of others and the mind and soul of universal Nature. For always the effect of the supramental growth is to universalise the individual consciousness. As it makes us live, even in our individual vital movement and its relations with all around us, with the universal life, so it makes us think and feel and sense, although through an individual centre or instrument, with the universal mind and psychical being. This has two results of great importance.

First, the phenomena of the psychical sense and mind lose the fragmentariness and incoherence or else difficult regulation and often quite artificial order which pursues them even more than it pursues our more normal mental activities of the surface, and they become the harmonious play of the universal inner mind and soul in us, assume their true law and right forms and relations and reveal their just significances. Even on the mental plane one can get by the spiritualising of the mind at some realisation of soul oneness, but it is never really complete, at least in its application, and does not acquire this real and entire law, form, relation, complete and unfailing truth and accuracy of its significances. And, secondly, the activity of the psychical consciousness loses all character of abnormality, of an exceptional, irregular and even a perilously supernormal action, often bringing a loss of hold upon life and a disturbance or an injury to other parts of the being. It not only acquires its own right order within itself but its right relation with the physical life on one side and with the spiritual truth of being on the other and the whole becomes a harmonious manifestation of the embodied spirit. It is always the originating supermind that contains within itself the true values, significances and relations of the other parts of our being and its unfolding is the condition of the integral possession of our self and nature.

The complete transformation comes on us by a certain change, not merely of the poise or level of our regarding conscious self or even of its law and character, but also of the whole substance of our conscious being. Till that is done, the supramental consciousness manifests above the mental and psychical atmosphere of being—in which the physical has already become a subordinate and to a large extent a dependent method of our self's expression,—and it sends down its power, light, and influence into it to illumine it and transfigure. But only when the substance of the lower consciousness has been changed, filled potently, wonderfully transformed, swallowed up as it were into the greater energy and sense of being, *mahān, br.hat,* of which it is a derivation and projection, do we have the perfected, entire and constant supramental consciousness. The substance, the conscious ether of being in which the mental or psychic consciousness and sense live and see and feel and experience is something subtler, freer, more plastic than that of the physical mind and sense. As long as we are dominated by the latter, psychical phenomena may seem to us less real, hallucinatory even, but the more we acclimatise ourselves to the psychical and to the ether of being which it inhabits, the more we begin to see the greater truth and to sense the more spiritually concrete substance of all to which its larger and freer mode of experience bears witness. Even, the physical may come to seem to itself unreal and hallucinatory—but this is an exaggeration and new misleading exclusiveness due to a shifting of the centre and a change of action of the mind and sense—or else may seem at any rate less powerfully real. When, however, the psychical and physical experiences are well combined in their true balance, we live at once in two complementary worlds of our being each with its own reality, but the psychical revealing all that is behind the physical, the soul view and experience taking precedence and enlightening and explaining the physical view and experience. The supramental transformation again changes the whole substance of our consciousness; it brings in an ether of greater being, consciousness, sense, life, which convicts the psychical also of insufficiency and makes it appear by itself an incomplete reality and only a partial truth of all that we are and become and witness.

All the experiences of the psychical are accepted and held up indeed in the supramental consciousness and its energy, but they are filled with the light of a greater truth, the substance of a greater spirit. The psychical consciousness is first supported and enlightened, then filled and occupied with the supramental light and power and the revealing intensity of its vibrations. Whatever exaggeration, whatever error born of isolated incidence, insufficiently illumined impression, personal suggestion, misleading influence and intention or other cause of limitation or deformation interferes in the truth of the mental and psychical experience and knowledge, is revealed and cured or vanishes, failing to stand in the light of the self-truth—*satyam, ṛtam*—of things, persons, happenings, indications, representations proper to this greater largeness. All the psychical communications, transcriptions, impresses, symbols, images receive their true value, take their right place, are put into their proper relations. The psychical intelligence and sensation are lit up with the supramental sense and knowledge, their phenomena, intermediate between the spiritual and material worlds, begin to reveal automatically their own truth and meaning and also the limitations of their truth and significance. The images presented to the inner sight, hearing, sensation of all kinds are occupied by or held in a larger and more luminous mass of vibrations, a greater substance of light and intensity which brings into them the same change as in the things of the physical sense, a greater totality, precision, revealing force of sense knowledge carried in the image. And finally all is lifted up and taken into the supermind and made a part of the infinitely luminous consciousness, knowledge and experience of the supramental being, the Vijnana Purusha.

The state of the being after this supramental transformation will be in all its parts of consciousness and knowledge that of an infinite and cosmic consciousness acting through the universalised individual Purusha. The fundamental power will be an awareness of identity, a knowledge by identity,—an identity of being, of consciousness, of force of being and consciousness, of delight of being, an identity with the Infinite, the Divine, and with all that is in the Infinite, all that is the expression and manifestation of the Divine. This awareness and knowledge will use as its means and instruments a spiritual vision of all that the knowledge by identity can found, a supramental real idea and thought of the nature of direct thought vision, thought hearing, thought memory that reveals, interprets or represents to the awareness the truth of all things, and an inner truth speech that expresses it, and finally a supramental sense that provides a relation of contact in substance of being with all things and persons and powers and forces in all the planes of existence.

The supramental will not depend on the instrumentation, for example, of the sense, as the physical mind is dependent on the evidence of our senses, although it will be capable of making them a starting-point for the higher forms of knowledge, as it will also be capable of proceeding directly through these higher forms and making the sense only a means of formation and objective expression. The supramental being will transform at the same time and take up into itself the present thinking of the mind transfigured into an immensely larger knowledge by identity, knowledge by total comprehension, knowledge by intimate perception of detail and relation, all direct, immediate, spontaneous, all the expression of the self's already existent eternal knowledge. It will take up, transform, supramentalise the physical sense, the sixth sense capacities of the mind and the psychic consciousness and senses and use them as the means of an extreme inner objectivisation of experience. Nothing will be really external to it, for it will experience all in the unity of the cosmic consciousness which will be its own, the unity of being of the infinite which will be its own being. It will experience matter, not only gross matter but the subtle and the most subtle, as substance and form of the spirit, experience life and all kinds of energy as the dynamics of the spirit, supramentalised mind as a means or channel of knowledge of the spirit, supermind as the infinite self of knowledge and power of knowledge and Ananda of knowledge of the spirit.

# TOWARDS THE SUPRAMENTAL TIME VISION

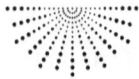

ALL BEING, consciousness, knowledge moves, secretly for our present surface awareness, openly when we rise beyond it to the spiritual and supramental ranges, between two states and powers of existence, that of the timeless Infinite and that of the Infinite deploying in itself and organising all things in time. These two states are opposed to and incompatible with each other only for our mental logic with its constant embarrassed stumbling around a false conception of contradictions and a confronting of eternal opposites. In reality, as we find when we see things with a knowledge founded on the supramental identity and vision and think with the great, profound and flexible logic proper to that knowledge, the two are only coexistent and concurrent status and movement of the same truth of the Infinite. The timeless Infinite holds in itself, in its eternal truth of being, beyond this manifestation, all that it manifests in Time. Its time consciousness too is itself infinite and maintains in itself at once in a vision of totalities and of particularities, of mobile succession or moment sight and of total stabilising vision or abiding whole sight what appears to us as the past of things, their present and their future.

The consciousness of the timeless Infinite can be brought home to us in various ways, but is most ordinarily imposed on our mentality by a reflection of it and a powerful impression or else made present to us as something above the mind, something of which it is aware, towards which it lifts, but into which it cannot enter because itself lives only in the time sense and in the succession of the moments. If our present mind untransformed by the supramental influence tries to enter into the timeless, it must either disappear and be lost in the trance of Samadhi or else, remaining awake, it feels itself diffused in an Infinite where there is perhaps a sense of supra-physical space, a vastness, a boundless extension of consciousness, but no time self, time movement or time order. And if then the mental being is still mechanically aware of things in time, it is yet unable to deal with them in its own manner, unable to establish a truth relation between the timeless and things in time and unable to act and will out of its indefinite Infinite. The action that then remains possible to the mental Purusha is the mechanical action of the instruments of the Prakriti continuing by force of old impulsion and habit or continued initiation of past energy, *prārabdha,* or else an action chaotic, unregulated, uncoordinated, a confused precipitate from an energy which has no longer a conscious centre.

The supramental consciousness on the other hand is founded upon the supreme consciousness of the timeless Infinite, but has too the secret of the deployment of the infinite Energy in time. It can either take its station in the time consciousness and keep the timeless infinite as its background of supreme and original being from which it receives all its organising knowledge, will and action, or it can, centred in its essential being, live in the timeless but live too in a manifestation in time which it feels and sees as infinite and as the same Infinite, and can bring out, sustain and develop in the one what it holds supernally in the other. Its time consciousness therefore will be different from that of the mental being, not swept helplessly on the stream of the moments and clutching at each moment as a stay and a swiftly disappearing standpoint, but founded first on its eternal identity beyond the changes of time, secondly on a simultaneous eternity of Time in which past, present and future exist together for ever in the self-knowledge and self-power of the Eternal, thirdly, in a total view of the three times as one movement singly and indivisibly seen even in their succession of stages, periods, cycles, last—and that only in the instrumental consciousness—in the step by step evolution of the moments. It will therefore have the knowledge of the three times, *trikāladṛṣṭi,*—held of old to be a supreme sign of the seer and the Rishi,—not as an abnormal power, but as its normal way of time knowledge. This unified and infinite time consciousness and this vision and knowledge are the possession of the supramental being in its own supreme region of light and are complete only on the highest levels of the supramental nature. But in the ascent of the human consciousness through the uplifting and transmuting evolutionary—that is to say, self-unveiling, self-developing, progressively self-perfecting—process of Yoga, we have to take account of three successive conditions all of which have to be overpassed before we are able to move on the highest levels. The first condition of our consciousness, that in which we now move, is this mind of ignorance that has arisen out of the inconscience and nescience of material Nature,—ignorant but capable of seeking for knowledge and finding it at least in a series of mental representations which may be made clues to the true truth and, more and more refined and illuminated and rendered transparent by the influence, the infiltration and the descent of the light from above, prepare the intelligence for opening to the capacity of true knowledge. All truth is to this mind a thing it originally had not and has had to acquire or has still to acquire, a thing external to it and to be gathered by experience or by following certain ascertained methods and rules of enquiry, calculation, application of discovered law, interpretation of signs and indices. Its very knowledge implies an antecedent nescience; it is the instrument of Avidya.

The second condition of consciousness is potential only to the human being and gained by an inner enlightening and transformation of the mind of ignorance; it is that in which the mind seeks for its source of knowledge rather within than without and becomes to its own feeling and self-experience, by whatever means, a mind, not of original ignorance, but of self-forgetful knowledge. This mind is conscious that the knowledge of all things is hidden within it or at least somewhere in the being, but as if veiled and forgotten, and the knowledge comes to it not as a thing acquired from outside, but always secretly there and now remembered and known at once to be true,—each thing in its own place, degree, manner and measure. This is its attitude to knowledge even when the occasion of knowing is some external experience, sign or indication, because that is to it only the occasion and its reliance for the truth of the knowledge is not on the external indication or evidence but on the inner confirming witness. The true mind is the universal within us and the individual is only a projection on the surface, and therefore this second state of consciousness we have either when the individual mind goes more and more inward and is always consciously or subconsciously near and sensitive to the touches of the universal mentality in which all is contained, received, capable of being made manifest, or, still more powerfully, when we live in the consciousness of universal mind with the personal mentality only as a projection, a marking board or a communicating switch on the surface.

The third state of consciousness is that of the mind of knowledge in which all things and all truths are perceived and experienced as already present and known and immediately available by merely turning the inner light upon it, as when one turns the eye upon things in a room already known and familiar,—though not always present to the vision because that is not attentive,—and notes them as objects of a pre-existent knowledge. The difference from the second self-forgetful state of consciousness is that there is here no effort or seeking needed but simply a turning or opening of the inner light on whatever field of knowledge, and therefore it is not a recalling of things forgotten and self-hidden from the mind, but a luminous presentation of things already present, ready and available. This last condition is only possible by a partial supramentalising of the intuitive mentality and its full openness to any and every communication from the supramental ranges. This mind of knowledge is in its essentiality a power of potential omnipotence, but in its actual working on the level of mind it is limited in its range and province. The character of limitation applies to the supermind itself when it descends into the mental level and works in the lesser substance of mentality, though in its own manner and body of power and light, and it persists even in the action of the supramental reason. It is only the higher supramental Shakti acting on its own ranges whose will and knowledge work always in a boundless light or with a free capacity of illimitable extension of knowledge subject only to such limitations as are self-imposed for its own purposes and at its own will by the spirit.

The human mind developing into supermind has to pass through all these stages and in its ascent and expansion it may experience many changes and various dispositions of the powers and possibilities of its time consciousness and time knowledge. At first man in the mind of ignorance can neither live in the infinite time consciousness nor command any direct and real power of the triple time knowledge. The mind of ignorance lives, not in the indivisible continuity of time, but successively in each moment. It has a vague sense of the continuity of self and of an essential continuity of experience, a sense of which the source is the deeper self within us, but as it does not live in that self, also it does not live in a true time continuity, but only uses this vague but still insistent awareness as a background, support and assurance in what would otherwise be to it a constant baseless flux of its being. In its practical action its only support other than its station in the present is the line left behind by the past and preserved in memory, the mass of impressions deposited by previous experience and, for the future, an assurance of the regularity of experience and a power of uncertain forecast founded partly upon repeated experience and well-founded inference and partly on imaginative construction and conjecture. The mind of ignorance relies on a certain foundation or element of relative or moral certainties, but for the rest a dealing with probabilities and possibilities is its chief resource.

This is because the mind in the Ignorance lives in the moment and moves from hour to hour like a traveller who sees only what is near and visible around his immediate standpoint and remembers imperfectly what he has passed through before, but all in front beyond his immediate view is the unseen and unknown of which he has yet to have experience. Therefore man in his self-ignorance moving in time exists, as the Buddhists saw, only in the succession of thoughts and sensations and of the external forms present to his thought and sense. His present momentary self is alone real to him, his past self is dead or vanishing or only preserved in memory, result and impression, his future self is entirely non-existent or only in process of creation or preparation of birth. And the world around him is subject to the same rule of perception. Only its actual form and sum of happenings and phenomena is present and quite real to him, its past is no longer in existence or abides only in memory and record and in so much of it as has left its dead monuments or still survives into the present, the future is not yet at all in existence.

It must be noted however that if our knowledge of the present were not limited by our dependence on the physical mind and sense, this result would not be altogether inevitable. If we could be aware of all the present, all the action of physical, vital, mental energies at work in the moment, it is conceivable that we would be able to see their past too involved in them and their latent future or at least to proceed from present to past and future knowledge. And under certain conditions this might create a sense of real and ever present time continuity, a living in the behind and the front as well as the immediate, and a step farther might carry us into an ever present sense of our existence in infinite time and in our timeless self, and its manifestation in eternal time might then become real to us and also we might feel the timeless Self behind the worlds and the reality of his eternal world manifestation. In any case the possibility of another kind of time consciousness than we have at present and of a triple time knowledge rests upon the possibility of developing another consciousness than that proper to the physical mind and sense and breaking our imprisonment in the moment and in the mind of ignorance with its limitation to sensation, memory, inference and conjecture.

Actually man is not content solely with living in the present, though it is that he does with the most pressing vividness and insistence: he is moved to look before and after, to know as much as he can of the past and try to penetrate as far as he can, however obscurely, into the future. And he has certain aids towards this endeavour of which some depend on his surface mind, while others open to intimations from another subliminal or superconscient self which has a greater, subtler and more certain knowledge. His first aid is that of the reason proceeding forward from cause to effect and backward from effect to cause, discovering the law of energies and their assured mechanic process, assuming the perpetual sameness of the movements of Nature, fixing her time measures and thus calculating on the basis of a science of general lines and assured results the past and the future. A certain measure of limited but sufficiently striking success has been gained by this method in the province of physical Nature and it might seem that the same process might eventually be applied to the movements of mind and life and that at any rate this alone is man's one reliable means in any field of looking with precision back and forwards. But as a matter of fact the happenings of vital and still more of mental nature escape to a very great degree the means of inference and calculation from assured law that apply in the field of physical knowledge: it can apply there only to a limited range of regularised happenings and phenomena and for the rest leaves us where we were amid a mixed mass of relative certainties, uncertain probabilities and incalculable possibilities.

This is because mind and life bring in a great subtlety and intricacy of movement, each realised movement carries in it a complex of forces, and even if we could disengage all these, all, that is to say, that are simply actualised and on or near the surface, we should still be baffled by all the rest that is obscure or latent,—concealed and yet potent contributory causes, hidden motion and motive force, undeployed possibilities, uncalculated and incalculable chances of variation. It ceases to be practicable here for our limited intelligence to calculate accurately and with certitude as in the physical field from precise cause to precise effect, that is to say, from a given apparent set of existing conditions to an inevitable resultant of subsequent or a necessary precedence of antecedent conditions. It is for this reason that the predictions and previsions of the human intelligence are constantly baffled and contradicted by the event, even when largest in their view of the data and most careful in their survey of possible consequence. Life and mind are a constant flux of possibles intervening between spirit and matter and at each step bring in, if not an infinite, at least an indefinite of possibles, and this would be enough to make all logical calculation uncertain and relative. But in addition there reigns behind them a supreme factor incalculable by human mind, the will of the soul and secret spirit, the first indefinitely variable, fluid and elusive, the second infinite and inscrutably imperative, bound, if at all, only by itself and the Will in the Infinite. It is therefore only by going back from the surface physical mind to the psychic and spiritual consciousness that a vision and knowledge of the triple time, a transcendence of our limitation to the standpoint and view range of the moment, can be wholly possible.

Meanwhile there are certain doors opening from the inner on to the outer consciousness which make an occasional but insufficient power of direct retro-vision of the past, circumvision of the present, prevision of the future even in the physical mind at least potentially feasible. First, there are certain movements of the mind sense and the vital consciousness that are of this character—of which one kind, that which has most struck our perceptions, has been called presentiment. These movements are instinctive perceptions, obscure intuitions of the sense mind and the vital being, and like all that is instinctive in man have been suppressed, rendered rare or discredited as unreliable by the engrossing activity of the mental intelligence. If allowed a free scope, these could develop and supply data not available to the ordinary reason and the senses. But still they would not be of themselves perfectly useful or reliable indices unless their obscurity were enlightened by an interpretation and guidance which the ordinary intelligence cannot give, but a higher intuition could provide. Intuition, then, is the second and more important possible means available to us, and actually intuition can and does sometimes give us in this difficult field an occasional light and guidance. But acting in our present mentality it is subject to the disadvantage that it is uncertain in operation, imperfect in its functioning, obscured by false imitative movements of the imagination and fallible mental judgment and continually seized on and alloyed and distorted by the normal action of mind with its constant liability to error. The formation of an organised intuitive mentality purified from these deficiencies would be needed to enlarge and assure this possibility of the functioning of a higher luminous intelligence.

Man, confronted by this incapacity of the intelligence and yet avid of the knowledge of the future, has fallen back on other and external means, omens, sortileges, dreams, astrology and many other alleged data for a past and future knowledge that have been in less sceptical times formulated as veridical sciences. Challenged and discredited by the sceptical reason these still persist in attracting our minds and hold their own, supported by desire and credulity and superstition, but also by the frequent though imperfect evidence we get of a certain measure of truth in their pretensions. A higher psychical knowledge shows us that in fact the world is full of many systems of correspondences and indices and that these things, however much misused by the human intelligence, can in their place and under right conditions give us real data of a supraphysical knowledge. It is evident, however, that it is only an intuitive knowledge that can discover and formulate them,—as it was in fact the psychical and intuitive mind that originally formulated these ways of veridical knowledge,—and it will be found in practice that only an intuitive knowledge, not the mere use either of a traditional or a haphazard interpretation or of mechanical rule and formula, can ensure a right employment of these indices. Otherwise, handled by the surface intelligence, they are liable to be converted into a thick jungle of error.

The true and direct knowledge or vision of past, present and future begins with the opening of the psychical consciousness and the psychical faculties. The psychical consciousness is that of what is now often called the subliminal self, the subtle or dream self of Indian psychology, and its range of potential knowledge, almost infinite as has been pointed out in the last chapter, includes a very large power and many forms of insight into both the possibilities and the definite actualities of past, present and future. Its first faculty, that which most readily attracts attention, is its power of seeing by the psychical sense images of all things in time and space. As exercised by clairvoyants, mediums and others this is often, and indeed usually, a specialised faculty limited though often precise and accurate in action, and implies no development of the inner soul or the spiritual being or the higher intelligence. It is a door opened by chance or by an innate gift or by some kind of pressure between the waking and the subliminal mind and admitting only to the surface or the outskirts of the latter. All things in a certain power and action of the secret universal mind are represented by images—not only visual but, if one may use the phrase, auditory and other images,—and a certain development of the subtle or psychical senses makes it possible,—if there is no interference of the constructing mind and its imaginations, if, that is to say, artificial or falsifying mental images do not intervene, if the psychical sense is free, sincere and passive,—to receive these representations or transcriptions with a perfect accuracy and not so much predict as see in its correct images the present beyond the range of the physical sense, the past and the future. The accuracy of this kind of seeing depends on its being confined to a statement of the thing seen and the attempt to infer, interpret or otherwise go beyond the visual knowledge may lead to much error unless there is at the same time a strong psychical intuition fine, subtle and pure or a high development of the luminous intuitive intelligence.

A completer opening of the psychical consciousness leads us far beyond this faculty of vision by images and admits us not indeed to a new time consciousness, but to many ways of the triple time knowledge. The subliminal or psychic self can bring back or project itself into past states of consciousness and experience and anticipate or even, though this is less common, strongly project itself into future states of consciousness and experience. It does this by a temporary entering into or identification of its being or its power of experiencing knowledge with either permanences or representations of the past and the future that are maintained in an eternal time consciousness behind our mentality or thrown up by the eternity of supermind into an indivisible continuity of time vision. Or it may receive the impress of these things and construct a transcriptive experience of them in the subtle ether of psychical being. Or it may call up the past from the subconscious memory where it is always latent and give it in itself a living form and a kind of renewed memorative existence, and equally it may call up from the depths of latency, where it is already shaped in the being, and similarly form to itself and experience the future. It may by a kind of psychical thought vision or soul intuition—not the same thing as the subtler and less concrete thought vision of the luminous intuitive intelligence—foresee or foreknow the future or flash this soul intuition into the past that has gone behind the veil and recover it for present knowledge. It can develop a symbolic seeing which conveys the past and the future through a vision of the powers and significances that belong to supraphysical planes but are powerful for creation in the material universe. It can feel the intention of the Divine, the mind of the gods, all things and their signs and indices that descend upon the soul and determine the complex movement of forces. It can feel too the movement of forces that represent or respond to the pressure—as it can perceive the presence and the action—of the beings of the mental, vital and other worlds who concern themselves with our lives. It can gather on all hands all kinds of indications of happenings in past, present and future time. It can receive before its sight the etheric writing, *ākāśa lipi*, that keeps the record of all things past, transcribes all that is in process in the present, writes out the future.

All these and a multitude of other powers are concealed in our subliminal being and with the waking of the psychical consciousness can be brought to the surface. The knowledge of our past lives,—whether of past soul states or personalities or scenes, occurrences, relations with others,—of the past lives of others, of the past of the world, of the future, of present things that are beyond the range of our physical senses or the reach of any means of knowledge open to the surface intelligence, the intuition and impressions not only of physical things, but of the working of a past and present and future mind and life and soul in ourselves and others, the knowledge not only of this world but of other worlds or planes of consciousness and their manifestations in time and of their intervention and workings and effects on the earth and its embodied souls and their destinies, lies open to our psychical being, because it is close to the intimations of the universal, not engrossed only or mainly with the immediate and not shut up into the narrow circle of the purely personal and physical experience.

At the same time these powers are subject to this disadvantage that they are not by any means free from liability to confusion and error, and especially the lower ranges and more outer workings of the psychical consciousness are subject to dangerous influences, strong illusions, misleading, perverting and distorting suggestions and images. A purified mind and heart and a strong and fine psychical intuition may do much to protect from perversion and error, but even the most highly developed psychical consciousness cannot be absolutely safe unless the psychical is illumined and uplifted by a higher force than itself and touched and strengthened by the luminous intuitive mind and that again raised towards the supramental energy of the spirit. The psychical consciousness does not derive its time knowledge from a direct living in the indivisible continuity of the spirit and it has not to guide it a perfect intuitive discrimination or the absolute light of the higher truth consciousness. It receives its time perceptions, like the mind, only in part and detail, is open to all kinds of suggestions, and as its consequent range of truth is wider, more manifold too are its sources of error. And it is not only that which was but that which might have been or tried and failed to be that comes to it out of the past, not only that which is but that which may be or wishes to be that crowds on it from the present and not only things to be but suggestions, intuitions, visions and images of many kinds of possibility that visit it from the future. And always too there is the possibility of mental constructions and mental images interfering with the true truth of things in the presentations of the psychical experience.

The coming of the intimations of the subliminal self to the surface and the activity of the psychical consciousness tend to turn the mind of ignorance, with which we begin, increasingly though not perfectly into a mind of self-forgetful knowledge constantly illuminated with intimations and upsurgings from the inner being, *antarātman*, rays from the still concealed awareness of its whole self and infinite contents and from the awareness—representing itself here as a sort of memory, a recalling or a bringing out—of an inherent and permanent but hidden knowledge of past, present and future that is always carried within itself by the eternal spirit. But embodied as we are and founded on the physical consciousness, the mind of ignorance still persists as a conditioning environment, an intervening power and limiting habitual force obstructing and mixing with the new formation or, even in moments of large illumination, at once a boundary wall and a strong substratum, and it imposes its incapacities and errors. And to remedy this persistence the first necessity would seem to be the development of the power of a luminous intuitive intelligence seeing the truth of time and its happenings as well as all other truth by intuitive thought and sense and vision and detecting and extruding by its native light of discernment the intrusions of misprision and error.

All intuitive knowledge comes more or less directly from the light of the self-aware spirit entering into the mind, the spirit concealed behind mind and conscious of all in itself and in all its selves, omniscient and capable of illumining the ignorant or the self-forgetful mind whether by rare or constant flashes or by a steady instreaming light, out of its omniscience. This all includes all that was, is or will be in time and this omniscience is not limited, impeded or baffled by our mental division of the three times and the idea and experience of a dead and no longer existent and ill-remembered or forgotten past and a not yet existent and therefore unknowable future which is so imperative for the mind in the ignorance. Accordingly the growth of the intuitive mind can bring with it the capacity of a time knowledge which comes to it not from outside indices, but from within the universal soul of things, its eternal memory of the past, its unlimited holding of things present and its prevision or, as it has been paradoxically but suggestively called, its memory of the future. But this capacity works at first sporadically and uncertainly and not in an organised manner. As the force of intuitive knowledge grows, it becomes more possible to command the use of the capacity and to regularise to a certain degree its functioning and various movements. An acquired power can be established of commanding the materials and the main or the detailed knowledge of things in the triple time, but this usually forms itself as a special or abnormal power and the normal action of the mentality or a large part of it remains still that of the mind of ignorance. This is obviously an imperfection and limitation and it is only when the power takes its place as a normal and natural action of the wholly intuitivised mind that there can be said to be a perfection of the capacity of the triple time knowledge so far as that is possible in the mental being.

It is by the progressive extrusion of the ordinary action of the intelligence, the acquiring of a complete and total reliance on the intuitive self and a consequent intuitivising of all the parts of the mental being that the mind of ignorance can be, more successfully, if not as yet wholly, replaced by the mind of self-contained knowledge. But,—and especially for this kind of knowledge,—what is needed is the cessation of mental constructions built on the foundation of the mind of ignorance. The difference between the ordinary mind and the intuitive is that the former, seeking in the darkness or at most by its own unsteady torchlight, first, sees things only as they are presented in that light and, secondly, where it does not know, constructs by imagination, by uncertain inference, by others of its aids and makeshifts things which it readily takes for truth, shadow projections, cloud edifices, unreal prolongations, deceptive anticipations, possibilities and probabilities which do duty for certitudes. The intuitive mind constructs nothing in this artificial fashion, but makes itself a receiver of the light and allows the truth to manifest in it and organise its own constructions. But so long as there is a mixed action and the mental constructions and imaginations are allowed to operate, this passivity of the intuitive mind to the higher light, the truth light, cannot be complete or securely dominate and there cannot therefore be a firm organisation of the triple time knowledge. It is because of this obstruction and mixture that that power of time vision, of back-sight and around-sight and foresight, which sometimes marks the illuminated mind, is not only an abnormal power among others rather than part of the very texture of the mental action, but also occasional, very partial and marred often by an undetected intermixture or a self-substituting intervention of error.

The mental constructions that interfere are mainly of two kinds, and the first and most powerfully distorting are those which proceed from the stresses of the will claiming to see and determine, interfering with knowledge and not allowing the intuition to be passive to the truth light and its impartial and pure channel. The personal will, whether taking the shape of the emotions and the heart's wishes or of vital desires or of strong dynamic volitions or the wilful preferences of the intelligence, is an evident source of distortion when these try, as they usually do try with success, to impose themselves on the knowledge and make us take what we desire or will for the thing that was, is or must be. For either they prevent the true knowledge from acting or if it at all presents itself, they seize upon it, twist it out of shape and make the resultant deformation a justifying basis for a mass of will-created falsehood. The personal will must either be put aside or else its suggestions must be kept in their place until a supreme reference has been made to the higher impersonal light and then must be sanctioned or rejected according to the truth that comes from deeper within than the mind or from higher above. But even if the personal will is held in abeyance and the mind passive for reception, it may be assailed and imposed on by suggestions from all sorts of forces and possibilities that strive in the world for realisation and come representing the things cast up by them on the stream of their will-to-be as the truth of past, present or future. And if the mind lends itself to these impostor suggestions, accepts their self-valuations, does not either put them aside or refer them to the truth light, the same result of prevention or distortion of the truth is inevitable. There is a possibility of the will element being entirely excluded and the mind being made a silent and passive register of a higher luminous knowledge, and in that case a much more accurate reception of time intuitions becomes possible. The integrality of the being demands however a will action and not only an inactive knowing, and therefore the larger and more perfect remedy is to replace progressively the personal by a universalised will which insists on nothing that is not securely felt by it to be an intuition, inspiration or revelation of what must be from that higher light in which will is one with knowledge.

The second kind of mental construction belongs to the very nature of our mind and intelligence and its dealing with things in time. All is seen here by mind as a sum of realised actualities with their antecedents and natural consequences, an indeterminate of possibilities and, conceivably, although of this it is not certain, a determining something behind, a will, fate or Power, which rejects some and sanctions or compels others out of many possibles. Its constructions therefore are made partly of inferences from the actual, both past and present, partly of a volitional or an imaginative and conjectural selection and combining of possibilities and partly of a decisive reasoning or preferential judgment or insistent creative will-intelligence that tries to fix among the mass of actuals and possibles the definitive truth it is labouring to discover or determine. All this which is indispensable to our thought and action in mind, has to be excluded or transformed before the intuitive knowledge can have a chance of organising itself on a sound basis. A transformation is possible because the intuitive mind has to do the same work and cover the same field, but with a different handling of the materials and another light upon their significance. An exclusion is possible because all is really contained in the truth consciousness above and a silencing of the mind of ignorance and a pregnant receptivity is not beyond our compass in which the intuitions descending from the truth consciousness can be received with a subtle or strong exactitude and all the materials of the knowledge seen in their right place and true proportion. As a matter of practice it will be found that both methods are used alternatively or together to effect the transition from the one kind of mentality to the other.

The intuitive mind dealing with the triple time movement has to see rightly in thought sense and vision three things, actualities, possibles and imperatives. There is first a primary intuitive action developed which sees principally the stream of successive actualities in time, even as the ordinary mind, but with an immediate directness of truth and spontaneous accuracy of which the ordinary mind is not capable. It sees them first by a perception, a thought action, a thought sense, a thought vision, which at once detects the forces at work on persons and things, the thoughts, intentions, impulsions, energies, influences in and around them, those already formulated in them and those in process of formation, those too that are coming or about to come into or upon them from the environment or from secret sources invisible to the normal mind, distinguishes by a rapid intuitive analysis free from seeking or labour or by a synthetic total view the complex of these forces, discerns the effective from the ineffective or partly effective and sees too the result that is to emerge. This is the integral process of the intuitive vision of actualities, but there are others that are less complete in their character. For there may be developed a power of seeing the result without any previous or simultaneous perception of the forces at work or the latter may be seen only afterwards and the result alone leap at once and first into the knowledge. On the other hand there may be a partial or complete perception of the complex of forces, but an incertitude of the definitive result or only a slowly arriving or relative certitude. These are stages in the development of the capacity for a total and unified vision of actualities.

This kind of intuitive knowledge is not an entirely perfect instrument of time knowledge. It moves normally in the stream of the present and sees rightly from moment to moment only the present, the immediate past and the immediate future. It may, it is true, project itself backward and reconstruct correctly by the same power and process a past action or project itself forward and reconstruct correctly something in the more distant future. But this is for the normal power of the thought vision a more rare and difficult effort and usually it needs for a freer use of this self-projection the aid and support of the psychical seeing.

Moreover it can see only what will arrive in the undisturbed process of the actualities and its vision no longer applies if some unforeseen rush of forces or intervening power comes down from regions of a larger potentiality altering the complex of conditions, and this is a thing that constantly happens in the action of forces in the time movement. It may help itself by the reception of inspirations that illumine to it these potentialities and of imperative revelations that indicate what is decisive in them and its sequences and by these two powers correct the limitations of the intuitive mind of actuality. But the capacity of this first intuitive action to deal with these greater sources of vision is never quite perfect, as must always be the case with an inferior power in its treatment of the materials given to it from a greater consciousness. A considerable limitation of vision by its stress on the stream of immediate actualities must be always its character.

It is possible however to develop a mind of luminous inspiration which will be more at home among the greater potentialities of the time movement, see more easily distant things and at the same time take up into itself, into its more brilliant, wide and powerful light, the intuitive knowledge of actualities. This inspired mind will see things in the light of the world's larger potentialities and note the stream of actuality as a selection and result from the mass of forceful possibles. It will be liable, however, if it is not attended with a sufficient revelatory knowledge of imperatives, to a hesitation or suspension of determining view as between various potential lines of the movement or even to a movement away from the line of eventual actuality and following another not yet applicable sequence. The aid of imperative revelations from above will help to diminish this limitation, but here again there will be the difficulty of an inferior power dealing with the materials given to it from the treasury of a higher light and force. But it is possible to develop too a mind of luminous revelation which taking into itself the two inferior movements sees what is determined behind the play of potentialities and actualities and observes these latter as its means of deploying its imperative decisions. An intuitive mind thus constituted and aided by an active psychic consciousness may be in command of a very remarkable power of time knowledge.

At the same time it will be found that it is still a limited instrument. In the first place it will represent a superior knowledge working in the stuff of mind, cast into mental forms and still subject to mental conditions and limitations. It will always lean chiefly on the succession of present moments as a foundation for its steps and successions of knowledge, however far it may range backward or forward,—it will move in the stream of Time even in its higher revelatory action and not see the movement from above or in the stabilities of eternal time with their large ranges of vision, and therefore it will always be bound to a secondary and limited action and to a certain dilution, qualification and relativity in its activities. Moreover, its knowing will be not a possession in itself but a reception of knowledge. It will at most create in place of the mind of ignorance a mind of self-forgetful knowledge constantly reminded and illumined from a latent self-awareness and all-awareness. The range, the extent, the normal lines of action of the knowledge will vary according to the development, but it can never be free from very strong limitations. And this limitation will give a tendency to the still environing or subconsciously subsisting mind of ignorance to reassert itself, to rush in or up, acting where the intuitive knowledge refuses or is unable to act and bringing in with it again its confusion and mixture and error. The only security will be a refusal to attempt to know or at least a suspension of the effort of knowledge until or unless the higher light descends and extends its action. This self-restraint is difficult to mind and, too contentedly exercised, may limit the growth of the seeker. If on the other hand the mind of ignorance is allowed again to emerge and seek in its own stumbling imperfect force, there may be a constant oscillation between the two states or a mixed action of the two powers in place of a definite though relative perfection.

The issue out of this dilemma is to a greater perfection towards which the formation of the intuitive, inspired and revelatory mind is only a preparatory stage, and that comes by a constant instreaming and descent of more and more of the supramental light and energy into the whole mental being and a constant raising of the intuition and its powers towards their source in the open glories of the supramental nature. There is then a double action of the intuitive mind aware of, open to and referring its knowledge constantly to the light above it for support and confirmation and of that light itself creating a highest mind of knowledge,— really the supramental action itself in a more and more transformed stuff of mind and a less and less insistent subjection to mental conditions. There is thus formed a lesser supramental action, a mind of knowledge tending always to change into the true supermind of knowledge. The mind of ignorance is more and more definitely excluded, its place taken by the mind of self-forgetful knowledge illumined by the intuition, and the intuition itself more perfectly organised becomes capable of answering to a larger and larger call upon it. The increasing mind of knowledge acts as an intermediary power and, as it forms itself, it works upon the other, transforms or replaces it and compels the farther change which effects the transition from mind to supermind. It is here that a change begins to take place in the time consciousness and time knowledge which finds its base and complete reality and significance only on the supramental levels. It is therefore in relation to the truth of supermind that its workings can be more effectively elucidated: for the mind of knowledge is only a projection and a last step in the ascent towards the supramental nature.

## ALSO BY SRI AUROBINDO

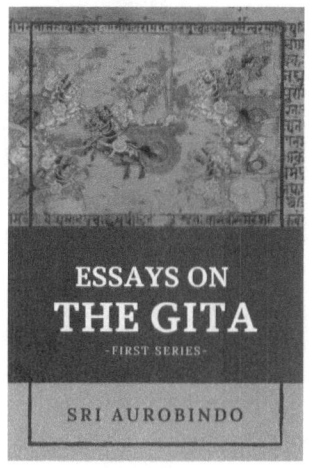

ESSAYS ON THE GITA

### FIRST SERIES

- ISBN PAPERBACK: 9782357286313
- ISBN HARDCOVER: 9782357286320
- ISBN E-BOOK: 9782357286337

### SECOND SERIES

- ISBN PAPERBACK: 9782357286481
- ISBN HARDCOVER: 9782357286498
- ISBN E-BOOK: 9782357286504

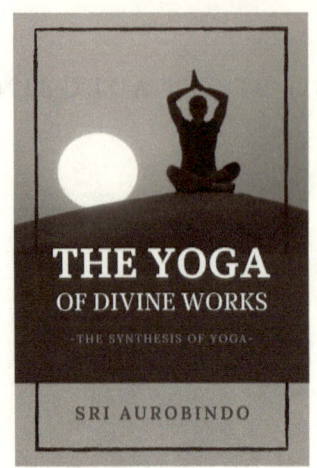

### THE YOGA OF DIVINE WORKS

- ISBN PAPERBACK: 9782357286511
- ISBN HARDCOVER: 9782357286528
- ISBN E-BOOK: 9782357286535

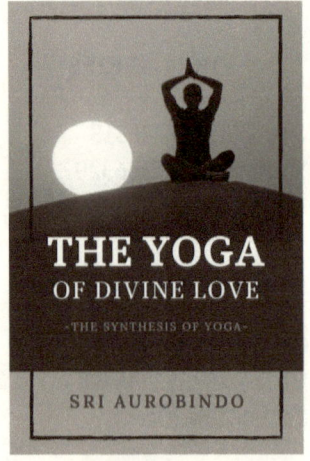

### THE YOGA OF DIVINE LOVE

- ISBN PAPERBACK: 9782357286870
- ISBN HARDCOVER: 9782357286887
- ISBN E-BOOK: 9782357286894

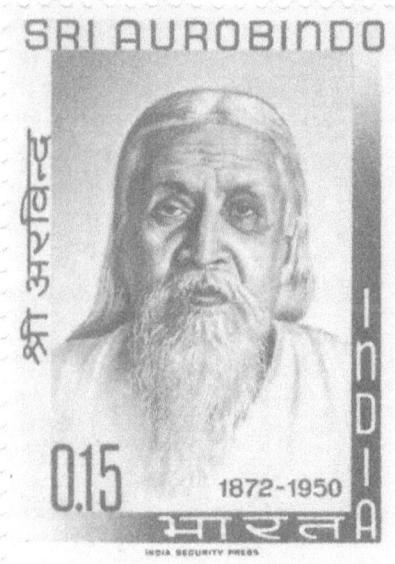

Copyright © 2021 by ALICIA EDITIONS
Credits: Canva
All rights reserved.
No part of this book may be reproduced in any form or by any electronic or mechanical means, including information storage and retrieval systems, without written permission from the author, except for the use of brief quotations in a book review.

www.ingramcontent.com/pod-product-compliance
Lightning Source LLC
LaVergne TN
LVHW040136080526
838202LV00042B/2931